T5-CCX-734

Irma Shorell

with Julie Davis

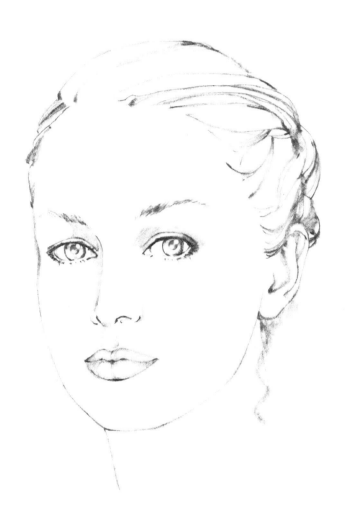

Illustrated by Elaine Yabroudy

A Lifetime of Skin Beauty: The Irma Shorell Program

SIMON AND SCHUSTER   NEW YORK

Published by Simon and Schuster
A Division of Gulf & Western Corporation
Simon & Schuster Building
Rockefeller Center
1230 Avenue of the Americas
New York, New York 10020
SIMON AND SCHUSTER and colophon are trademarks of Simon & Schuster

Designed by Elizabeth Woll

Manufactured in the United States of America

10   9   8   7   6   5   4   3   2

Library of Congress Cataloging in Publication Data
Shorell, Irma.
       A lifetime of skin beauty.

       1. Skin—Care and hygiene.   2. Beauty, Personal.
I. Davis, Julie,   II. Title.
RL87.S53   646.7′26   81–13632
ISBN 0–671–42274–X   AACR2

FOR TIM

*the most compassionate, lovable and
lively person I ever knew*

FOR TIM

*the most compassionate, lovable and
lively person I ever knew*

I wish to acknowledge my father, Dr. I. Daniel Shorell, who helped me to start a whole new life with one jar of cream. My love and gratitude go to those who work with me, my husband, Hal Lightman, our partner, Harry Steinfield, Kathy Cappiello and Gene Barnes. And to my daughter, Stacey, our teen adviser, and her brother, Chip, for his input on the importance of skin care for men.

I want to thank all the leading plastic surgeons and dermatologists who helped me, especially Dr. Jane Haher who graciously donated her time and expertise in the field of cosmetic plastic surgery for our chapter on this always fascinating subject; Catherine Shaw, our editor, whose enthusiasm and meticulous editing made the book come alive; and Cris Alexander for his wonderful photographs.

IRMA SHORELL

I wish to acknowledge my father, Dr. I. Daniel Shorell, who helped me to start a whole new life with one jar of cream. My love and gratitude go to those who work with me, my husband, Hal Lightman, our partner, Harry Steinfield, Kathy Cappiello and Gene Barnes. And to my daughter, Stacey, our teen adviser, and her brother, Chip, for his input on the importance of skin care for men.

I want to thank all the leading plastic surgeons and dermatologists who helped me, especially Dr. Jane Haher who graciously donated her time and expertise in the field of cosmetic plastic surgery for our chapter on this always fascinating subject; Catherine Shaw, our editor, whose enthusiasm and meticulous editing made the book come alive; and Cris Alexander for his wonderful photographs.

IRMA SHORELL

Contents

PART I

Formula for Beauty

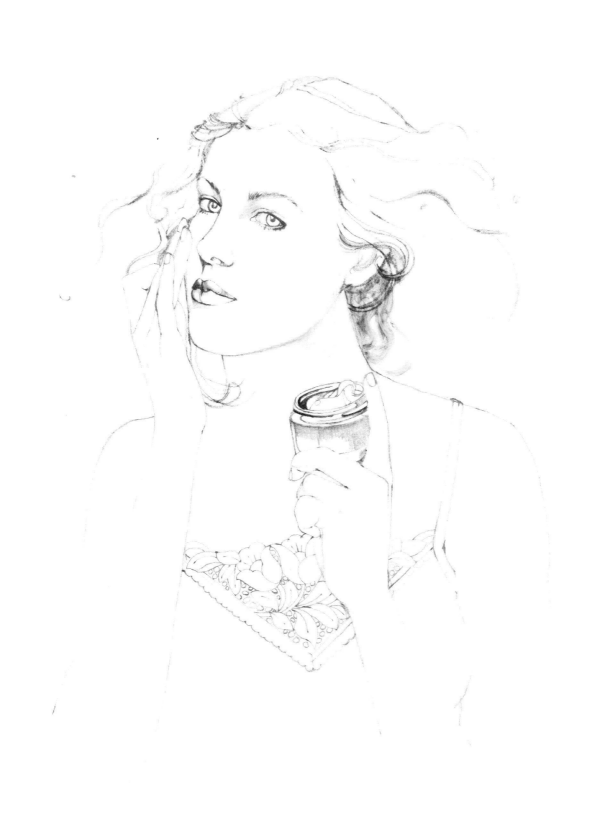

CHAPTER 1

"Can I Be Beautiful?" My Most Frequently Asked Question

Y<small>ES!</small>

That's a question that has always interested me. The desire to be beautiful—we all share it, women across the country, across the globe. I can't remember a time when I wasn't conscious of my appearance, doubly so when I felt I didn't look my best and found myself face to face with a ravishing lady. But I knew—even before I became involved in the business of being beautiful twenty years ago—that even the most attractive woman wasn't born that way. She achieved her perfection by enhancing her best features, her eyes, her lips and, most of all, her complexion. (The born beauty isn't as lucky as we think: while an awkward teen can turn herself into a stunning thirty, the girl who blossoms at eighteen and doesn't bother to learn how to maintain her looks won't enjoy as pretty a future!) *Beauty is in the hands of every woman who wants it.*

Ever since Max Factor and Technicolor, women have been more intrigued by the magic of makeup than by the basics of skin care. Fortunately, in the eighties we now know that beauty doesn't come from a tube of foundation, and that no makeup can do its best job unless you start with clear, healthy skin that's scrupulously clean. To that end, finding the most effective skin-care system is the number one priority. And the American woman spends close to a billion dollars a year trying to do just that!

But products and preparations are only secondary to more practical principles that cost only a little thought and that will encourage real beauty—the kind you literally create from within. Just as exercise builds a firm, strong body that lets you throw away your lingerie foundations, caring for your skin will enable you to cast off your makeup foundation and, if you care for it well, all but one of your beauty cremes. I don't think you'll find many cosmetic manufacturers ready to admit that, but it's true.

The beauty formula I'm asked for by the women I meet in stores, on airplanes and via my talk shows is based on five sound principles that you can start practicing right away, before you reach for your favorite moisturizer, and certainly before you spend another dollar on the next "miracle" product to be touted about town. Here they are—don't lose another minute.

1. Water Is Your First Beauty Basic

A favored gimmick on many jars of beauty creme is the word "natural," but when you study the label carefully you see that, more often than not, water is the only natural ingredient the creme contains. Water is a fabulous cleanser and has great therapeutic value—the well-known spas of the world all know this.

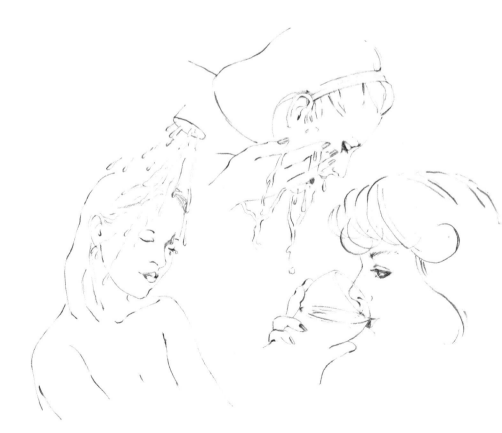

Water is as valuable to you inside as out. Drinking eight glasses of water a day cleanses the internal system and replenishes the normal fluid balance (the body is 80 percent water and up to two quarts a day are lost through natural body functions). Used with a liquid cleanser, there's no beauty lotion more efficient. Splash it on with calculated abandon to stimulate the pores—use first warm, then cool water, but never extremely hot or cold. No more need for toners or fresheners or, for those with oily skin, astringents.

People often disagree about what kind of water to use: tap water, bottled spring water, imported waters. I believe that's a matter of personal choice, but you should know that research is showing our own tap water as having better than adequate purity; the water in New York is rated among the highest in taste and wholesomeness.

2. A Daily Skin-Care Plan Is a Must— But Keep It Simple

Clear, healthy skin is skin that is cared for, well cleansed and lubricated. But achieving it never has to be a chore. For me, seven minutes in the morning and seven minutes at night is all the time I need. My plan is ideal for the busy woman—in a word: uncomplicated. I cleanse my face and neck, rinse with warm, then cool, water, pat dry and apply my moisturizer first thing in the morning; at night, after cleansing and stimulating, I finish with a nourishing creme, a slightly denser formula than the moisturizer, as my skin tends to be dry. And that's it. Nothing could be simpler.

Complicated skin-care routines aren't better; they're a bother. After two or three days, they're about as exciting as cleaning the kitchen floor! And those women who think of extra time spent as pampering them-selves should know that overtreating your complexion can cause as many problems as outright neglect. Dab on all sorts of preparations and you can find yourself with a serious case of clogged pores. I don't believe in spending hours in the bathroom giving my skin a work-over.

Of course, some women have special complexion problems (ex-cessive dryness or aggravated acne, to name only two) that call for the attention of a dermatologist, or at least some extra care. I'll tell you more about effective solutions for these and other woes later on.

One caution: you'll be tempted to pat yourself on the back once you put my plan into effect—but don't become discouraged if you **don't** see overnight results. Most of us want instant gratification and, when disappointed, give up too soon. Patience, as well as dedication, is needed —and rewarded.

3. A Little Makeup Goes a Long Way

When I was in my twenties and interested in looking older, I got into the habit of the "full face" (foundation, powder, blushers) until I realized that this was indeed aging me, and in two ways—neither of which I wanted! First, makeup settles into the skin, exaggerating and eventually deepening even the finest lines of dry areas, and clogging and congesting the enlarged pores of oily areas. Second, makeup suffocates

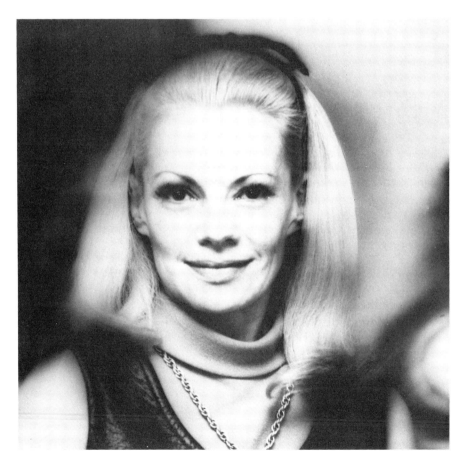

the skin, impeding its "breathing" of oxygen needed to abet a healthy tone.

Another drawback to makeup is the difficulty of removing it, especially if, at the end of a long day, you do nothing more than cream off surface impurities. That's just not enough. You haven't freed the pores of makeup pigments and daily soil. If you must wear foundation, you'll have to deep-cleanse nightly with equal dedication.

I'm not suggesting that you stop wearing cosmetics altogether— but you should be more selective about those you do use. I've stopped using foundation and powder, and only occasionally do I wear blusher. Though I'm the first to acknowledge its many wonderful uses, you'd be surprised at the glow you can achieve through skin care alone. I agree with the cosmetics companies that an effortless, natural look is most appealing, but we part company when they contradict themselves by telling you how to *paint it on!* All you need to do is bring out your own inborn beauty by taking advantage of your complexion's eager responsiveness. That way the only beautifiers you'll need are mascara and lipstick—and won't that be a boon to your cluttered cosmetics case!

4. Develop Your Sunsense

Solar energy is terrific, but the sun's effects on the complexion make it Public Enemy Number One. Next to chronological aging, it is the single greatest cause of premature lines and a loss of the skin's youth-preserving elasticity—damage that won't get moisturized away. Overexposure can mean as few as ten unprotected minutes if you have fair skin and light hair. Dry, leathery skin is one result; skin cancers are another. Who needs either?

Most people think of the sun only in summer, but whether you're poolside, downhill racing or driving in your car, even on a cloudy day, the sun is busy at work—working on you! Of course, you can't spend your life hiding out, but you can take preventive measures to keep your skin soft and dewy.

Sun blocks and screens limit the sun's harmful ultra-violet rays, letting you savor outdoor activities all year long; the right sports gear will also protect; extra at-home care compensates for all environmental ravages: cold, high humidity, an arid climate, even indoor air conditioning and steam heat. Precautions are the answer, because it is far easier to prevent skin problems than to correct them.

5. Maintain a Supportive System for Skin Beauty

Why is it that every year you make, and break, the same promises? Proper eating habits, adequate rest and a healthy dose of exercise are always on the list (particularly after a wild New Year's Eve!), but all too soon forgotten. Yet these three elements are the keys to a healthy body and a healthy complexion. Start getting ready today for next December 31.

Your diet nourishes every part of you from within—and that includes each layer of your skin. Because I believe in that tried-and-true saying, *You are what you eat*, I make sure to have plenty of fresh fruits and vegetables as part of my daily intake.

Exercise promotes stamina and good circulation, which increases the flow of nourishing blood and its oxygen to your skin. A twice-a-week exercise class combined with a quick at-home stretch every morning keeps my body humming.

Sleep gives your system a well-deserved break from the stress of daily life and gives your face a rest from smiling, talking, eating, laughing, squinting—all the facial expressions that make lines. Too many late nights can result in dark circles under the eyes, sallow skin and lethargy, that tired, rundown feeling that dampens your mood and your looks. Sleep is the one beauty treatment that takes no effort, so get your rest to look your best. (Even when I don't get the eight hours that I need, I'm sure to compensate the following day with a short nap or a few minutes with my legs propped up—great for the circulation.)

The last part of your support system is harder to practice—making yourself happy. A renowned New York dermatologist once told me that happiness is the best medicine. To prove his point, he added that he has never had to treat a prospective bride. Of course, there are few times as ecstatic as your wedding day and you can't wash morning and night with a bottle of happiness (that's one formula I'd love to develop!), but you can enhance the quality of your personal life. That's as important for your state of mind as for your looks. Any negative emotion—stress, anxiety, impatience—shows readily on your face: you not only feel blue, you look blue, and those expression lines become a part of you, even when your mood changes.

Developing a positive outlook becomes even more invaluable as we get older. I'm a firm believer in guarding against wrinkles, but it is high time we stopped worrying about every little line—they just can't be put off forever. Yes, looking twenty-two is lovely, but once it's gone, there's no use bemoaning it—the only thing that can really make you look old is the idea that you are old. In the past two decades, middle age has shifted upward: we're living longer and we should be thinking young longer. As I see it, that choice is to our advantage.

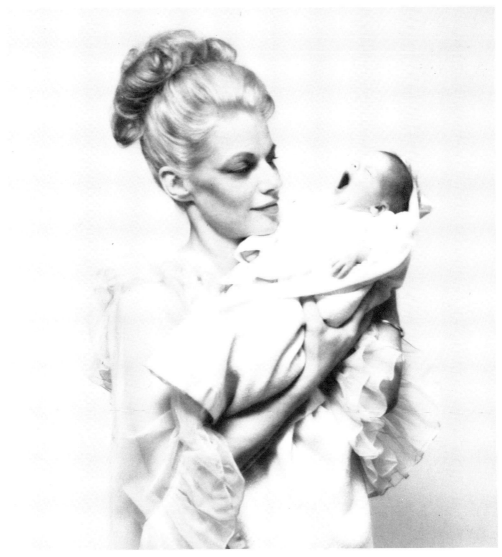

I've always said that life begins at forty. When I had my third child, Stacey, I felt that even my skin had a new start on life.

These are the principles I follow and recommend, and they come before any beauty products, even my own. In fact, unless you adopt this beauty know-how, you won't see the results you want, even if you're using the best skin-care line available.

THE MYTH OF THE MIRACLE

To achieve every goal in life, you have to be willing to expend a little effort. Becoming beautiful is no exception. The results will come from you, not any miracle product. The "miracle diet" that lets you eat anything you want doesn't work (unless you're trying to *gain* weight). Those "miracle exercise pants" that claim to sweat off your excess don't work (those are vital body fluids you're losing, not fat). That new jar of "miracle creme" will never make you look twenty years younger—even plastic surgery can't go that far, unless you're ninety-two and want to look seventy-two again!

It's time to put the effects of skin-care products, effective as these may be, back into perspective. No jar will turn back the clock, no matter how expensive: mine can't, *theirs* can't. There are no overnight sensations.

I know that's not what you want to hear—I certainly didn't. But I found out that accepting this sad fact is the first step in the only surefire way to succeed at being beautiful: a thorough, no-nonsense approach to skin, one that will start working to preserve your assets and even improve them.

Each of my five principles is detailed in the many chapters of this book. You'll learn enough about yourself to be the best judge of what's good for you. But first I'd like to share with you the path that led to my discoveries—how I, like so many women, had let myself go, and how developing my own approach (and starting my own skin-care business) helped me find my way back to beauty so that today I'm proud to admit I'm fifty-five!

CHAPTER 2

Skin Care:
A Shorell Family Enterprise

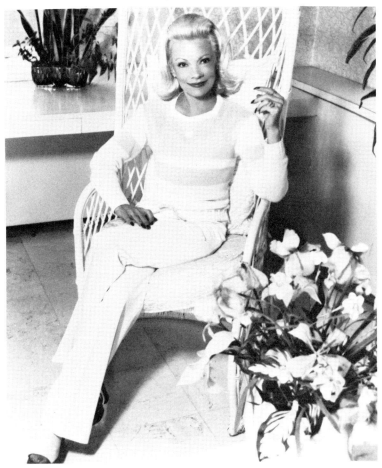

Lᴵᴷᴱ most mothers, I started my daughter Stacey on her beauty course. But I learned about beauty from my *father!* Dad was Dr. I. Daniel Shorell, a pioneer in the field of reconstructive and cosmetic plastic surgery and a firm believer in preventive skin care. He prescribed a proper "diet" for the skin, just as he advocated a correct, sensible diet for the whole body. He'd always say, "The basis of all facial beauty is a good skin. Good skin must be clean—clean deep down." In fact, he once confided to me that he thought he'd have about 10 percent fewer patients if only people would cleanse thoroughly every night. I knew early on that cleansing the face and neck was of the utmost importance —more important than the makeup I was nonetheless anxious to try. My problem would be to find the best products to do that job. I didn't know it when I was growing up, but my father had developed not only the beauty knowledge every woman needs, but also the beautifiers, *one* cleanser and *one* creme that would not only make me a part of that spared 10 percent, but also would land me smack in the middle of one of the most fascinating industries of the world, the business of beauty. And beauty was something I have always been very aware of.

Because my father's practice catered to the rich and the famous and because so many of them became friends of our family, I grew up in an aura of glamour and mystery, surrounded by beautiful women, or women on their way to being beautiful, often for the second time. Having a facelift was a carefully guarded secret in the forties and fifties; there was something hush-hush about it, especially when a patient traveled to my father's private hospital in New York from abroad. She (or *he*) would recuperate in one of the grandly appointed suites of the townhouse on East Seventy-first Street just off Fifth Avenue—my father would often invite his patients to our home. Seeing women wearing dark glasses whether to hide their identity or post-operative evidence of cosmetic surgery (sutures and the like), became less and less a novelty. Before I was old enough to wear lipstick, I was aware of age and of every woman's desire to look younger once she passed twenty-five!

Looking back, I believe there was probably too much emphasis placed on good looks at my house; but it's a fact of life that our first attraction to one another is physical—we put a lot of stock in appearance. Father was simply able to do something about it for his patients. But what I admired even more than his skill was his dedication. Though much of his (unwanted) publicity came from his "café society" patients (whose right to privacy he always tried to protect by denying any professional association with them), he was always available to those who needed surgery for reasons far more important than vanity. His doors were open to those whose very life depended on reconstructive surgery—from RAF pilots who couldn't chance the delicate procedures during the wartime bombings in London to victims of the great Texas

City fire of 1947, to those who came to his free clinics with seemingly irreparable congenital or accident-related disfigurements.

I best remember my father's story of how he had met and married my mother while studying at Georgetown Medical School, and how he had set up his practice with little money to speak of. He would tell my sister Joan and me how early he had left home to seek his fortune—the last time I think his age had dwindled down to twelve. Actually, he was such a remarkable man that I doubt that was all that far from the truth. His career has remained my inspiration.

Thankfully, Dad believed in bringing his work home with him, making me very conscious of my appearance—so much so that despite my petite size, I enjoyed my first career as a model. At fifteen, while still attending the Gardiner School, I posed for talented artist Dora— one of her imaginative sketches hangs proudly in my office. After graduation, it was on to Saks Fifth Avenue, where I modeled bathing suits: my small stature worked to my advantage! (At the time, taller girls were thought to look too "undressed" in swim suits.)

Three years later, I made my first venture into the world of cosmetics. Well, let's say I was lured in. I was having my hair done at my favorite salon, the House of Blondes, then located on East Sixty-first Street. The salon featured a makeup artist who had her private-label cosmetics manufactured for her. Impressed with my looks and my manner, she approached me and asked if I'd like to be her assistant. She needed a right hand so that she could open concessions at other salons about town. My parents were still in New York (Dad would soon move his hospital to Miami) and I wasn't too concerned about salary since I was living at home. Fine, I said and before my hair was dry, I had a smock around me and a makeup brush in my hand. I was quite excited.

I can't say the same for my first client however. I learned how to put mascara on another person—the hard way! But I had a wonderful teacher and I picked up her makeup tricks quickly; that, coupled with my past experimenting with friends, soon had me in demand for weddings and the like. After a few weeks, I was a real pro. My boss did very well too—her name is Estée Lauder.

Estée had a wonderful manner; she mesmerized women with her lovely complexion and her savvy. Patrons were eager to use her creme while under the dryer; as it melted away their makeup, they would ask her to apply her own cosmetics, and invariably Estée made a sale. She was a pro, very businesslike and with lots of ambition. She deserves the success and recognition she has today.

After that year-long fling with makeup, I studied dramatic art, doing a few years of summer stock, taking classes with Eli Wallach, landing a few small parts. I was thrilled to join Actors Equity, only to realize that breaking into the business was so tough, you received a pair of shoes along with your membership card. At the time, giving up my acting stint for a third career, wife and mother, was the best role I could ask for.

Taking care of my husband, H. Allen (Hal) Lightman, and my two young sons, Tim and Chip, kept me quite busy—far busier than I had realized. Out of the limelight, I grew less aware of my looks. Where was the time? What complicated the physical strain that was ravaging my complexion was not having a satisfying treatment system to use. I hadn't forgotten my father's beauty basics, but, now in my thirties, basic white soap and cold cream were no longer enough. And yet, there wasn't anything around better than soap and water. I had always felt lucky about my skin: I didn't have any of the usual adolescent problems such as acne; my freckles seemed to go with being petite. In my twenties and early thirties, during my two pregnancies, I'd been in great shape; the hormonal activity made my skin glow. But I found out that pregnancy is not a skin-care plan you can use continually. Caring for two small, active boys was depleting my reserves—and my complexion. Looking in the mirror one morning, I was shocked at the lines forming around my mouth and the corners of my eyes, at the dryness and poor color and tone of my skin. I knew I needed a rest, and I took a trip to Florida to visit my father.

One startled look from the doctor confirmed my own diagnosis— I needed help. Somehow, hearing how I looked from my own father sent the message home far more clearly. He told me that if my looks kept deteriorating I'd be wanting him to give me a facelift in fifteen years, but, he added, he wouldn't be able to do as good a job as I could do myself if I was willing to start right away and maintain the program. To accomplish this bit of preventive medicine, he gave me a jar of creme he had developed for his patients to tone the skin and keep the contours firm. This worked for both his post-operative patients and those he felt could forestall a facelift with extra care and attention.

Plastic-surgery techniques were so new in my father's day, and having the procedures done for purely cosmetic reasons even more so, that no post-operative products had been developed, much less marketed. Dad felt the need for such a creme and he worked out a formula of his own. Because it was given only to his patients and not commercially prepared, it was very thick and not very pretty or aromatic. But it worked! My father explained to me that surgery can remove loose skin that has sagged (partially because of neglect); but it cannot improve the quality of the skin or its color, or make surface lines disappear. The creme helped these problems.

I began using the preparation once a day, after cleansing, simply applying it before bed. After using it faithfully for three weeks, I began to see an improvement in my looks. Friends began to notice, too. Knowing that my father was a plastic surgeon, some even hinted that maybe I had had a facelift. When they found out the truth, they pleaded with me for some of the creme. Soon I had Dad sending so many jars that I jokingly said to my husband, Hal, we ought to be selling it. I told my father he really had a true-to-life beauty secret in his little jars. They both told me I was crazy. Fortunately for me, that was all the prompting I needed to plunge right in.

Actually, two things conspired to make me take that plunge. Most importantly, I liked the creme and its effects on my skin—I would never have thought of marketing a product I didn't believe in, because it would be impossible for me to tout it. And secondly, having always worked at exciting jobs, I was fairly frustrated at being home all the time. Though no one can deny that caring for two children is a career in itself, I was certain I could be a two-career woman. I had often helped out at the advertising agency my husband and his partner, Harry Steinfield, started after working together at the Amos Parrish agency— moonlighting after their business day was over became so profitable that they had struck out on their own, full time. Now I wanted something of my own.

I started by convincing Hal and Harry to give me space in the office (I quickly put up a bright yellow sheet to partition off my area), by convincing Dad to give me the formula, and by convincing myself to take my fifteen hundred dollars in savings and risk it on the venture. I knew this was the hardest task I had ever set for myself, but I knew also it would be better to try and fail than not to attempt it at all. What I never imagined was that refining the creme itself—improving the consistency of what was a less-than-attractive heavy pink substance— would be the most difficult of all.

My father gave me his formula on the condition that he wouldn't have to be involved with its promotion. In those days the American Medical Association didn't want its physicians and surgeons attracting any more publicity (read: notoriety) than was necessary. My father liked being a part of the AMA and he didn't want to jeopardize his good standing. (Today doctors can't wait to get on TV for the publicity, but then you didn't even allow your name in the newspapers, much less advertise your successful patients and operations!) But Dad did insist that certain criteria be met. Foremost in his mind was that the creme be formulated by a pharmaceutical company. The creme isn't based on any "miracle" ingredient; its effectiveness is due, rather, to the way in which its ingredients are compounded. My father refused to entrust this crucial procedure to a cosmetics lab, no matter how well recommended.

Because the creme itself had to meet my approval as well as the doctor's, it took more than a year to achieve a product that was satisfactory to us all. Dad wanted to be sure his original formula was followed. Looking at it from the point of view of the customer, I wanted it to be cosmetically acceptable. But we all were concerned with insuring its lasting effectiveness. You see, after Dad blended a batch, he would give it directly to his patient. But the route from the pharmaceutical company to a store's shelf is more roundabout. Our creme had to be ready, in jars, when we received orders. The jars would then be placed on a truck, often ill-ventilated and hot, and be transported over great distances. More often than not, the jars would go not directly to the store but to the store's consolidator, a vast receiving warehouse, like one of those on the West Side docks in Manhattan. It might take two or three days to sort them out from among dresses or bed linens, making the entire journey anywhere from two to ten days! Afterward, the jars might sit on the store shelf for up to a month until they were all sold. Hopefully every store rotates its stock, selling the last jar or two of a previous shipment before it sells the new ones, but it can happen that those last jars get hidden behind the new stock, and are sold months later.

No one can indefinitely guarantee a product, especially a creme, but like all other manufacturers, we wanted one that would stay fresh as long as possible, long after it was brought home. Too, everyone has harmless organisms that live on the body, but once you use your finger to apply a product, you introduce those organisms to the product, and often they don't get along. My creme had to include a preservative to inhibit their proliferation and further insure the creme's effectiveness.

All these factors combined to increase the difficulty of getting the creme ready. I remember how hard it was to get just the right consistency —sometimes it was too thick, other times too thin, or the creme didn't go on well, or I just didn't like the feel of it. The first samples I was pleased with were shipped to Florida for my father's approval—and promptly vetoed for one reason or another. I'll never forget watching over a batch as it was being stirred by a giant oar and thinking to myself, Why isn't it ready yet?

After much waiting, our creme was perfected and named "Formula M7." To insure a consistently first-quality product, every batch would be tested by me or one of our experts—that's still true today.

The next step was packaging, a very crucial element—the package itself had to have great appeal. And this is where Hal and Harry's advertising know-how saved the day. We all agreed on the look we wanted—very serious and highly ethical, no fluff, nothing that looked like anything else available. At the time the trend was toward pastels, lots of pink, white, light-blue boxes. We opted for a mysterious square black box! The jar for the creme itself was chosen as carefully: a stylish footed jar, with just a bit of a shape, a rounded bottom. It bore a simple label designed to look just like the one you'd see on a prescription item —a doctor's prescription on that beautiful opaque glass jar.

There was just one slight problem. We found that our shiny black paper label, chosen because it resisted becoming dog-eared on the shelf, also resisted all kinds of ink! We wanted luxurious engraving done in white but found nothing to adhere to the glossy coating of the paper.

Well, we were undaunted in those days, and I called on all the top printers, determined to start with the letter A and go all the way to Z to find someone who could do the job. A lot of inks were formulated for me, but none worked. By a great stroke of luck, Harry discovered an oldtime engraver working out of the smallest shop in the Wall Street area—he was easily in his eighties, maybe even his nineties. He scratched his head when confronted with the situation, the black paper and the multitude of white inks I had in my possession. He asked for a little time to ponder the dilemma and within a couple of weeks had developed his own ink that took to the paper. By now I was sure I was on the right track.

So much of my money had been spent already that it was impossible to have the boxes professionally wrapped. Hal and I would cover them with cellophane ourselves—I'd frequently tape Hal's fingers to the package. Despite this and his initial skepticism, he was beginning to share my enthusiasm. Along with Harry, we did everything ourselves— except, thankfully, to make the creme on the kitchen stove.

I was lucky to have the agency's support and the help of a handful of others who spread the Shorell message. Hal had the idea for me to run single-column ads that looked more like editorials—they were eye-catching and they worked—so well that I still use this format today.

The late Helen Van Slyke, who later achieved her greatest fame as the author of many best-selling novels, was, before her literary career, both an advertising copywriter and a buyer at New York's Henri Bendel. Helen wrote the first store advertisement based on Hal's idea.

I knew that I wanted to be selective about the stores I sold to and I liked the idea of selling to Bendel—that name had the cachet I wanted for my product. Bendel, in turn, liked to premiere the finest in beauty and fashion, and being the first to feature Formula M7 appealed to them greatly. (Little did they know we were so exclusive that we often walked over from our Madison Avenue office and delivered their orders personally.) I was beginning to establish myself.

My first bit of publicity was a news story in *The New York Times*, based on a United Press wire-service story about M7 and the Shorell family. But what really put me on the map was the marvelous feature Eugenia Sheppard wrote in the *Herald Tribune*. It didn't take long for the famed columnist to make the connection between I.S. Laboratories (the company name listed on my product) and Dr. Shorell, the surgeon whose name, much to his chagrin, had been in the gossip columns since the forties. I will always be grateful to her—the spread opened the doors to the city's many influential beauty editors and beauty buyers across the country.

Neiman-Marcus in Texas was one of the next stores I sold to—in a very roundabout way. I had sent a sample to the cosmetics buyer, who was less than interested. But instead of sending back the creme, he gave it to one of the store's leading models, a very attractive woman in her forties who, like me, hadn't been satisfied by anything on the market. After using the creme for three weeks, the model went straight to Stanley Marcus to suggest that he carry the line. She was allergic to almost everything she had ever tried, but Formula M7 had worked for her. That buyer who had never heard of me suddenly became very enthusiastic too!

When that story was told to me, I had an idea I thought would make other buyers intrigued enough to try the creme in a more direct fashion. Along with my samples, I sent a letter suggesting that the cosmetic sales staff try Formula M7 for three weeks. If they weren't happy with it, I wouldn't ask for an order again. I was certain that if, on the other hand, they were satisfied with the results, they would be more interested in selling the product than if they were to sell it blind. Soon Saks Fifth Avenue and I. Magnin in California were active accounts. I was in business! (Today, I am pleased to be able to say that more cosmetic retailers themselves use my products than any others sold in their stores.)

Marketing Formula M7 was a triumph for me. I was proud of the role I had played in its development and I was determined to be a part of its continued success—which is why we have remained a family business. To really bring home my ideas on the personal approach, I thought it important to visit each of the stores that sold my product, to meet the buyers, the sales staff as well as the people in shipping and receiving. I learned about them and they learned more about me and Formula M7. I didn't realize at the time how grueling the road can be, or how many branches our largest chain, I. Magnin, had throughout California—and I was committed to visit each one. I would start with a little talk to the store gathering and most of my speech was impromptu, but I invariably began with "I can't tell you how pleased and proud I am to be here at I. Magnin in San Francisco" or ". . . I. Magnin in Santa Barbara." But one day, after having seen more branches than I could remember, I got as far as ". . . I. Magnin in—"and stopped short. I turned quickly to Hal and asked, "Where are we?"

I learned a lot about the beauty business and about the cities and towns of California on that trip!

Eventually, my nerves calmed and I got into the habit of jotting

I started my business with my father's formula, $1,500, a corner of Hal's office . . . and this fashionable outfit for my first personal appearances!

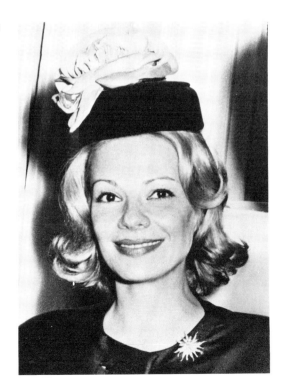

down little notes for myself before each appearance. Of course my acting training was a great preparation for me, especially when I began to do live TV talk shows and radio guest spots.

The traveling and the promoting were excellent for business. What had first been a handicap—having a skin-care line of *one* product—was adding to the Shorell mystique. At first, my chief worry had been getting enough counter space to be visible in the stores; in short order, I had to worry about whether or not the pharmaceutical company could produce our next 5,000-jar batch in time for reorders. They needed about six weeks to fill our order, making the timing very close—cautiously I had waited until the initial supply was half depleted before placing my second order.

Remembering the elation of opening that perfected first jar and seeing its lovely pink-peach color, I anxiously awaited the next ones. Well, the jars arrived at the office—still Hal and Harry's—and we all fell in a dead faint: the creme was a bright yellow!

Of course, I was convinced that the lab had sent the right jars filled with the wrong creme. And I was frantic—soon I'd be faced with orders I couldn't fill.

The pharmaceutical company had records of the various checks made at different stages of production and they showed that our formula had been compounded correctly, that the correct ingredients had been used. But how could this be? we all wondered. And then the production manager reminded us that my father had outlawed the use of any artificial coloring in the creme. All the ingredients were natural, and as natural ingredients can vary in color, so can the products they are used to formulate. He gave me an easy-to-understand example, too: the color of butter varies from bright yellow in summer to pale yellow in winter because cows eat grass in the warm months, straw or hay in the cooler ones.

I talked this over with my father, who felt it was just as simple (and far safer) to put an explanatory note in the packages as to add a coloring agent to his formula. Hal turned this minus into a plus by furthering Dad's reasoning: he had the instruction booklets reprinted, explaining the possible confusion over color changes and adding the advantages of a creme that is made as naturally as possible.

No more scares, but a lot of hard work went into the next two years as we built our reputation—and I increased the size of my make-shift office. There *was* one very mysterious incident—with a very funny ending. This happened at Saks Fifth Avenue.

Formula M7 was extremely well received in the four specialty stores in which it was first sold. In the sixties, a specialty store catered exclusively to women, and was the perfect forum for a creme designed for the very discerning. In its two-year history, no jar had ever been returned—a record that made me very pleased. So when we learned that a jar had been brought back to the Saks Fifth Avenue store, we all walked right over. I was very concerned about maintaining our quality standards; if something had gone awry, I wanted to know what it was.

The customer had sent back the jar three-quarters full, saying she thought something was wrong with it, asking for a replacement. I was ready to accommodate her when Miss Marian Combs, the pretty Scottish doyenne of the cosmetics department, who had been keeping her beauty counters spic and span since my modeling days at Saks, asked if she could look at the jar before it was sent to our lab for testing.

Thanks to Miss Marian, as the dear lady was fondly called, I received my first backhanded compliment. The creme had been three-quarters used, or emptied into another jar, only to be replaced with mashed potatoes veiled with a thin layer of M7 as a guise for the customer to get a free second jar! I was glad that we had yet another satisfied customer, but dumbfounded that she would go to such lengths for more. After that episode, I realized that a businesswoman has to be prepared for everything.

Far from being content to sit back and relax, I wanted to expand my line to include a good cleanser—after all, my old soap-and-water routine had contributed greatly to the waning of my looks. I again turned to my father and asked what he relied on. His surgical scrub, I learned. Could it be adapted for me? Yes. We removed the harsher ingredients needed to achieve a surgeon's degree of cleanliness (those that killed staph and other germs). I then had a two-product line that incorporated water, my first essential, as a rinse in between.

I was only one step away from completing a skin-care plan designed for the woman over thirty-five. Needed was a light creme that could easily be worn during the day, under makeup if desired, to offer some protection against the elements. At about this time we had decided to change the name of Formula M7 to Contour/35, a name we could copyright. Too many over-the-counter medicines were using the word "formula" and we felt that our creme's name should more accurately reflect the job it was designed to do: *Contour*, because it maintains the firm contours of the face; *35* because it answers the needs of women with mature (often prematurely dry) skin. Its companion product, I

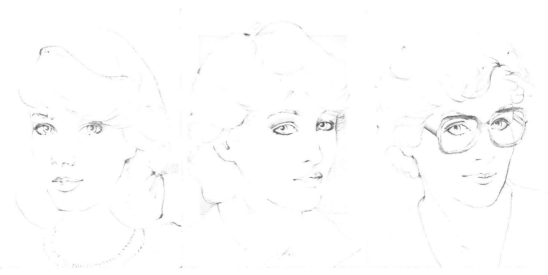

At each of the stages of your life, it's important to evaluate your skin's needs.

reasoned, should be a lighter formulation of the same basic ingredients, just as cologne is a lighter version of a perfume, with the same basic notes. So Moisture/35 was developed to moisturize the "over 35" complexion.

The Youth/25 version of my three-product line was conceived in the late sixties, when it occurred to me that if postponing signs of age after a woman reached her thirties worked, the regime would be even more effective if begun in her twenties. Using the two basic formulas for a creme and a cleanser, I brought out Youth/25 moisturizing creme, good day and night, and Youth/25 deep-acting facial cleanser to free young skin of excess oils and grime.

Not unlike our first attempts at adapting Formula M7, we had problems homogenizing this lighter version with its greater oil content. On the packages I explain that Youth/25 creme may be slightly grainy, often due to atmospheric conditions, and that it can easily be blended before use with its little applicator—far preferable to our adding a stabilizing agent. None of the letters we've received about it ever expressed any dissatisfaction. In fact, once, we had a letter quite to the contrary. It was from a woman who had been using it for ten years and had always found these "lumps" in it. But the last jar she bought she found perfectly blended, and she called us frantically, long distance, to beg us to put our *beauty grains* back in the formula!

My next skin-care product—the last one designed for the face, specifically—came about after I had a frightening mishap. While I was using one of the popular drain decloggers I accidently spilled some on my hand and then unwittingly touched it to my face. I mistakenly tried to wash off the last traces with water—finding out the hard way that this merely activated the powerful ingredients. I could practically hear my face sizzling—it was even more scary than it sounds! Well, the next morning, I found a patch like a dark scab on the side of my face and immediately called a friend who was a dermatologist. She explained that it would require a lengthy healing process for my skin to repair itself but that I could use a slightly abrasive cleansing pad and lotion daily to stimulate the appearance of new cells. This was a method she prescribed to patients with blackheads and poor circulation as well. The doctor

A skin-care emergency led me to develop my dermabrasing system to slough off dead skin cells and revivify the complexion.

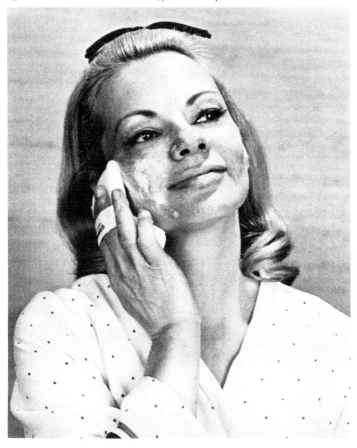

gave us the idea to develop our own lotion formula—we called it Dermabrase. I coined that word to describe the gentle abrasive action I achieved. Don't confuse it with dermabra*ding*, from the technique called dermabrasion, a medical treatment that attempts to drastically change the appearance of the skin through the use of harsh chemicals, and not always with the desired results. Mine is a gradual skin-renewal procedure—you won't see the radical results of surgery, but over a period of weeks, and without the risks, you will see clearer skin.

Like most women, I was concerned mostly with my facial appearance and barely thought below the neck. But once I had achieved the results I wanted for my complexion, I wanted silky soft skin all over. Bodybrase/35 was created for the rough skin of the elbows and knees (and the hips and thighs, if necessary). Its companion products—a bath oil, a foaming gel and a body lotion—followed.

Filling a need—for myself, Hal, the kids, our friends—that's really the way I created each of my products. My children, fair-haired and very susceptible to sunburns, were the reason I developed sun-care products, particularly a complete sun block that didn't wash off in the water, where the sun's rays can also penetrate. And I developed a creamy, easy to apply and tissue off eye-makeup remover only after I heard the complaints of dozens of women (cosmetics buyers among them) that, regardless of which brand of remover they had been using, they always woke to find pillowcases smudged with leftover remover and mascara.

I've never once thought to myself, Today, I'll experiment for something new. I'm not in the market to find that one revolutionary product—I don't think it exists. But when I see a need, that's when I go to work.

When I bring out a product, I'm not content to advertise it as "new"; I have to be able to say it's new *and it works*. I can stand behind each of my products because I have personally tested them for six months before making them available. My product line is still very small—that's because I don't think you need more than one cleanser, one creme, one body lotion. I don't make a special creme for the eye area or for the elbows or for the toenails like so many of my competitors do—they are unnecessary. I don't offer a selection of cleansers—things like a milky liquid, a creme you wipe off, a dissolving gel: all gimmicks. Just one basic cleanser in two forms, the mild version geared to the older woman, the more potent version for younger, oilier skin. Beauty doesn't have to be complicated or costly.

Today, with the Shorell name in over six hundred stores across the country and abroad, my main concern is maintaining a relationship with each and every one of the shops. The sales staff is my link to my customers, and because salesgirls change so often, it's a round-the-clock job to stay abreast of who's who.

Visiting a store is always a lot of fun, whether it's a giant like Macy's–California (one of the few *department* stores I'm in—that's how impressed I am with its luxury) or a select shop like Haddad's in Charleston, West Virginia, where I was greeted with great pomp and circumstance. My schedule in Charleston is a terrific example of my day on the road: a breakfast meeting with the staff, a presentation of my training program for the sales people, an informal chat with customers, interviews at the newspapers, an appearance on the local morning talk show—far from the nine-to-five life!

I suppose I have Hal and Harry to thank—they made me my own

I may have started out with only a corner in Hal's office—but today I have the corner suite, *complete with an exciting Manhattan view!*

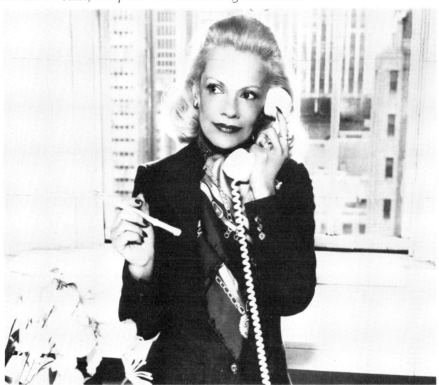

model, a position I've held for twenty years now. "Look at me if you want proof that my product works," was my slogan, and today it's still me the stores want.

If you're wondering about my husband and his partner—well, they eventually went to work for their biggest advertising account—me! Their success in advertising had been based on acquiring many small accounts. That way, they figured, losing one or two would never mean ruin. But as the Shorell name grew, as they dropped an account, they never bothered to replace it, taking more of a role in my company. I laugh now when I think of that tiny area I had in their old office, because in my new location I have the largest office of all. The funniest development is that Hal (who pleaded with me not to try my hand against the cosmetics companies) was so impressed with the line's effects on *his* skin that he adapted the line for men—and Shorell for Men is proving as successful as its forerunner. One of my happiest moments was when my son Chip, attending college in Miami, asked to be our representative to the stores in that area, meeting with buyers and taking care of our orders. He proved to have a good head for business.

I feel proud that I was a pioneer in the beauty business, in making my father's creme available to the public—heir to his pioneering in creating it along with his surgical procedures. And it's wonderful to think that my children may carry on our family's affair with beauty.

Are you listening, Stacey?

PART II

The Basics of Beautiful Skin

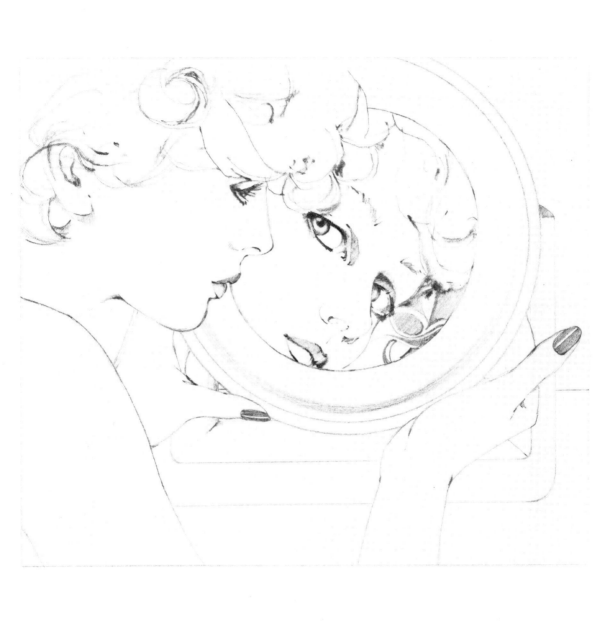

CHAPTER 3

Seven Minutes to a Lovelier Complexion

SKIN care is deceptively simple. My own plan takes only seven minutes in the morning and seven minutes at night. But if you use the wrong products—or the right products the wrong way—whether you take seven minutes, or seventy, you won't be doing yourself any good, and maybe even do some harm.

Understanding the role of skin care, knowing all about your complexion and learning the function of the basic skin-care products (the fewer the better) is very important. Following any skin-care strategy blindly—without knowing why you're following those steps—inevitably leads to disaster. So before I chart my seven-minute regimen for you, here's a basic primer on the skin, its role and its needs. It will probably take you longer to read this than to actually cleanse your complexion— but unlike cleansing, this is something you only need to do once, and it's more than worth the effort.

A Little Understanding

The skin is an amazing organ (yes, *organ*, and the body's largest— almost six pounds of your body weight!) and it responds fantastically to your care. Part of that small wonder is its great resiliency: skin can often heal itself after minor cuts and accidents, even from break-outs (if you stop squeezing and aggravating the condition). And a little attention—the right attention—satisfies its beauty needs.

The skin's most important functions, however, have nothing to do with beauty. As an envelope, it protects the body against cold and illness while sealing in vital fluids and shielding the underlying tissues from bruises. The body uses the skin to regulate internal temperature: the skin releases heat as perspiration, one of our most natural processes.

It has often been said that the skin is the barometer of the emotions: it blushes from embarrassment, pales from fear. Even more accurately, it reflects the state of the body. (A perfect example of this relationship occurs during the disease hepatitis. One of the first symptoms is jaundice, a yellowing of the skin.) Taking care of the body is the first priority for good health and the healthiest skin.

Bits of Biology

The skin is really two layers of activity working as one: the epidermis, or the skin's skin, and the dermis, the activity center replete with blood vessels, hair follicles (or roots), nerve endings and oil glands. The dermis is often called the "true" skin because its processes determine the quality of the epidermis. But because the epidermis, where the skin cells actually grow, mature and die (at the skin surface) is what we see, our beauty thinking often stops there.

The skin's *elasticity* is the factor that determines your complexion's "age appearance"—not how old your skin is, but how old it looks. My father explained this concept to me using a rubber band. When a baby is born, her skin is as elastic as the rubber band; after being stretched, it contracts to its original shape immediately. But as the child grows to be an adult, and as the adult ages, like the rubber band, stretched every day, the skin gets less and less elastic; it remains stretched out and limp, its flexibility is gone.

The idea is to sustain the skin's elasticity as long as possible: if you maintain this quality, the skin will work well, look well.

BEAUTY BASIC: *Don't sleep on your face—this distorts its natural shape, stretches the skin needlessly.*

BEAUTY BASIC: *Don't go on a roller coaster of rapid weight loss and gain. This stretches the skin, causing it to lose its resiliency, so that over a period of time it will no longer be able to contract after weight loss.*

BEAUTY BASIC: *Don't smoke. Pursing the lips causes lines around the mouth; the smoke causes squint lines around the eyes.*

The Fallacy of the Flawless Complexion

I'm not convinced that anyone has a flawless complexion by birth. Even that smooth, peaches-and-cream skin of certain women in their early twenties has its problems: it's a sensitive skin that can't go out in the sun, that reacts unpredictably to makeups, and that develops irritations at the drop of a hat even though to the outside world it *looks* great. The truly lucky woman is the one with very average skin: a bit oily, a bit more olive. This skin is much more tolerant of the elements and makeup and it stays youthful and moist longer. With the right care, it can be improved so that it looks great, too.

The Facts About Your Complexion

To improve your skin by way of skin-care products, these must be selected and used with regard to your complexion's unique characteristics. First, of course, you have to know what those characteristics are. That seems easy enough, but you'd be surprised at the small percentage of women who can accurately describe their complexion. Some like to classify skin by type: "normal," "oily," and "dry"—this technique should have gone out with the stone age: there is no such thing as normal skin, any more than there is one normal hair color or height. Others offer degrees of oiliness and dryness and that great euphemism for anything that doesn't fit either: the "combination" skin.

I prefer to forget about "types," and talk about needs, the little extras that individualize basic cleansing and care: the oily chin, the dryness under the eyes, etc. Instead of my giving you a random number of category choices and asking you to adjust yourself to one of them, I want you to devise your own complexion composition and chart your individual characteristics on the figure on page 45. First read the following Facial Profile to be alert to the most prevalent complexion conditions and then use the Skin Characteristics Charts on page 43 to detail each part of your face: the forehead and temples, the nose, the upper lip, the chin, the cheeks, the area around the eyes, the jawline and the neck. You'll then have, possibly for the first time, an exact picture of your complexion—and I do mean *yours*.

The Facial Profile

Every woman has a certain number of oil glands to nourish the face. The number may be small or large, but whatever you've got, they're concentrated in the center of the face, most often around the nose, frequently around the forehead and the chin as well—the infamous "T-zone." Unless your oil glands are gushing, the outer areas of the face, along the temples to the cheeks and down around the jawline to the neck, tend to be dry. The explanation is simple: the oils retain the body's vital fluids (what we commonly call moisture), and the resulting softness is lost to areas the oils don't reach.

There is nothing wrong with a light, dewy veil of the skin's natural oils—this stalls the signs of advancing age. The last thing you want to do is scour your oils away with harsh astringents. (However a shine is not the only thing the oily skin develops—it can easily develop pimples, especially when the oils are trapped beneath the surface, causing bumps rather than the blackheads that clog pore openings.) Very oily areas need to be controlled, especially during the teen years when oil production peaks.

All-over oiliness can continue indefinitely, possibly lessening with time. An oily T-zone and mildly oily patches can equalize in your twenties and thirties. But if the skin goes too far in this direction and starts losing too many oils, it becomes dry in any number of areas. Slightly dry areas need moisturizing; very dry areas need a hard-working creme. When? Your chronological age isn't so much a factor as the visual age of your skin, determined by such conditions as your living environment. For instance, a woman living in hot, dry El Paso, Texas, might look up to seven years older than she is (say, thirty rather than her real age of twenty-three) because of the climate—unless, of course, she begins using a moisturizing creme in her teens.

Past the age of thirty-five, the skin starts to lose its moisture at an increasing rate—and all too often you hasten this along. Staying out too long in the sun, keeping the airconditioner on too high and for too long—these weaken the skin's natural defenses, its tolerance to the elements and its ability to adjust itself. Especially vulnerable now on even the oiliest complexions is the skin around the eyes, the thinnest of the whole envelope,* with few, if any, oil glands supplying it. It is

---

* Over-all skin averages 1.2 millimeters (or 1/10 inch) in thickness; the skin of the eyelid is .5 millimeters, less than half that!

especially susceptible to lines, but I don't recommend an excess of care: gently apply your moisturizing creme in the morning, remove makeup carefully at night and keep from touching in between.

After fifty, the skin is dramatically different. Unpredictable hormonal changes can cause the sharpest decrease in oil secretions—the skin does not retain its moisture, losing its plumpness and elasticity if unprotected. A very oily complexion may, however, finally equalize itself—no longer either greasy or dry. Pay careful attention to the upper lip area, now prone to thin, vertical lines running toward the nostrils.

SKIN CHARACTERISTICS CHARTS

SIGNS OF OILINESS

- enlarged pores

- clogged pores: oils have hardened in the pore openings; tips of the blackheads are visible

- pimples: oils are trapped beneath the surface; area can be reddened, with no visible pore openings

- area becomes very shiny to greasy only 1 hour after cleansing

- dark skin tone: sallow to olive to brown color

- skin often tans easily

SIGNS OF DRYNESS

- fine, closed pores

- skin can be smooth to parched to rough

- no tacky shine, no pimples

- fine, thin lines that deepen with neglect over time

- light skin tone: ivory to pink skin color

- skin burns easily, often sensitive to products

- little tolerance to extreme weather: chaps, flakes easily

THE SENSITIVITY FACTOR

your skin is *sensitive* if it reacts to almost anything: different fabrics, a new makeup, any creme, the sun, fragrances; is often uncomfortable, unpredictable

your skin is *allergy-prone* if it reacts to a specific thing: a fruit, wool, an ingredient or chemical in particular (example: fish scales in iridescent powders)

SKIN DIFFERENTIALS:
OTHER FACTORS THAT INDIVIDUALIZE YOUR SKIN

Quality	Degree	How to Improve It
elasticity	you do not retain expression lines *or* you faintly retain them, *or* they're a part of you	lubrication: moisturizer and/or creme
texture	smooth *or* smooth areas *or* rough areas	gentle stimulation to remove those dead skin cells on the skin surface
tone	even *or* fairly even *or* blotchy	correct cleansing to free pores, encourage circulation, which enhances tone

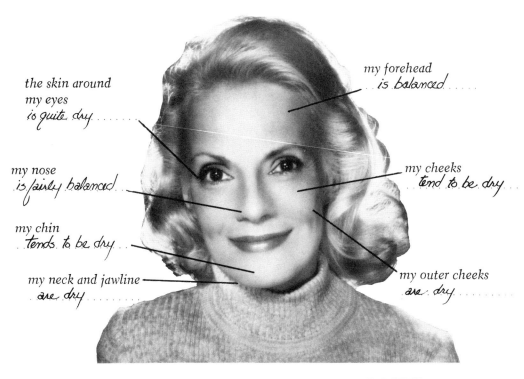

the skin around my eyes *is quite dry*

my nose *is fairly balanced*

my chin *tends to be dry*

my neck and jawline *are dry*

my forehead *is balanced*

my cheeks *tend to be dry*

my outer cheeks *are dry*

IRMA'S COMPLEXION COMPOSITE

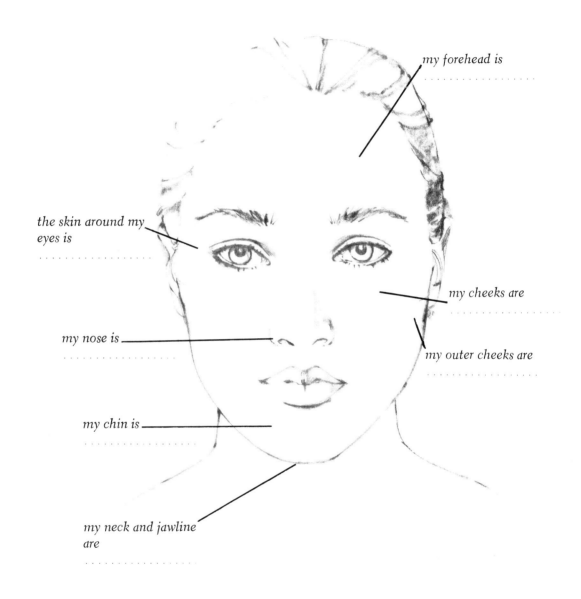

my forehead is
....

the skin around my
eyes is
....

my cheeks are
....

my nose is
....

my outer cheeks are
....

my chin is

my neck and jawline
are
....

YOUR COMPLEXION COMPOSITE

Your Facial Profile

Thoroughly cleanse your face, but don't apply anything after you've patted skin dry. Wait one hour, then in bright light (sunlight through a window, if possible) examine your face carefully in a mirror—a magnifying mirror will be helpful, if a bit frightening at first. Starting at your forehead, and working your way around your face, fill in all the blanks from the choices on the characteristics charts—one or two, any combination, maybe all. Remember to note your skin differentials, too. Armed with your composite, you can properly apply the needed products to the correct areas and work to balance your complexion.

The Results—The Best Incentive for Skin Care

I'm being realistic when I say that all the talk in the world about the good health of the body and the complexion won't get some people to wash their face. But mentioning the beauteous and lasting results may convince them—and encourage *you.*

You can see by reading the last of the characteristics charts that the skin's external qualities (its tone, its texture . . .) can be improved by skin care: cleansing, clarifying and lubricating. And that's not the only advantage of skin care: it discourages those signs of age we all fear by protecting the skin against wrinkle-forming elements like wind, cold and the sun.

Now that you know your own complexion's weaknesses—the areas that need your attention—adopt my three skin-care resolutions (don't wait until the New Year; do it today) and then *give yourself seven days to try my simplified plan.* Three weeks is the usual amount of time I keep a new product on trial when I'm testing the competition, but after only one week, I think you'll be satisfied enough to go on.

IRMA'S RESOLUTIONS

1. Promise never to go to sleep without removing your makeup and cleansing your face thoroughly!	2. Promise always to apply a good creme before retiring (don't forget your neck!)	3. Promise to observe this simple procedure · cleanse, · moisturize, · face the world every sun-up!

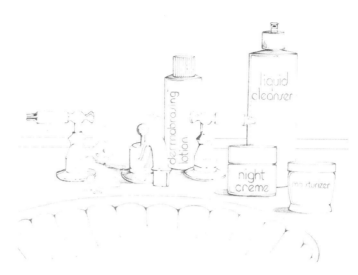

Pass the Products, Please!

As a businesswoman, I don't believe in the product-for-the-sake-of-product philosophy; I believe something is worthy only when it fills a need.

As a beauty consumer, I don't believe in buying a multitude of products. In fact, I like the idea of buying one product at a time, acclimating myself to it and only then incorporating a second component into my program. (In just this way, I started with my father's face creme and got used to it before I went on to use his scrub as my cleanser.) Most women don't want to bother with a dozen beauty aids. All too often the complicated routine is abandoned and the whole collection banished from the shelf as unsatisfactory mainly because they weren't given a fair try.

Though we all recognize the need for skin care, real interest in products is lacking on both the part of manufacturers and consumers. Cosmetics manufacturers go into this area because they know the financial rewards, but fail to bring to it the same dedication they give to makeup. Consumers allow themselves to be easily misled by their claims, which are thought up not by a scientist researching the given product, but by a clever ad agency executive. Everyone's fond of asking what's new and different. But I'm a firm believer in the question, What's old and still effective? With the proper advertising, you can sell anything—once. But if the product isn't effective, it won't sell again, especially if it broke too many promises. *Effective*—that's the most important quality you want from your skin-care tools: not the color, not the fragrance, not the empty promises.

The following is a list of the skin-care products that will meet the variety of needs your complexion composite indicates. Choose only the ones you need—one, two or more.

Note: I may lose some of the kitchen-as-a-beauty-source devotees, but I have to say that I don't believe in the "yogurt-Crisco" school of home remedies. Most food-based recipes are great—to eat! But don't put them on your face; the skin can't absorb their vitamins and nutrients. Your digestive track is what breaks food down into its components, and that's how you get the benefits. Banana-and-guava mash on your face will only get . . . moldy.

LIQUID CLEANSER

I love the clean feeling of soap-and-water washing—but it's not worth the dryness that follows. I use a liquid cleanser that is activated by water—it leaves my skin deep-down clean, without the harshness of ordinary soap made with detergents that remove needed moisture.

The formulation you choose should be especially gentle if you have dry skin. Like my Formula for Cleansing, it shouldn't contain any alkali or drying ingredients, but should have a softening lotion built in to leave skin smooth.

You need a deep-acting cleanser for oily skin because the oils frequently attract a lot of grime and leave a residue on your skin. My Youth/25 Facial Cleanser is a harder-working version of my father's formula, yet it isn't drying.

Beware of cleansing cremes that you have to tissue off—you need water for really effective cleansing (cremes leave a residue of oils mixed with skin's dirt and stale makeup; *alcohol-based cleansers* that wipe off dirt with cotton also wrongly omit the water step—and, because many applications may be needed until the cotton comes clean, you may be drying out your surface skin.

People use astringents thinking they will stop oil production—well, that process is a glandular one and nothing topical (applied to the surface) will change it. The astringent will, however, dry out the top layer of skin, trapping the oils under the surface. That spells P—I—M—P—L—E—s!

DERMABRASING LOTION

Provided you use an effective liquid and slightly abrasive applicator, this is a boon to sluggish skin that doesn't renew itself as quickly as you would like. Often, the top layer of skin cells (read: dead cells) hangs around just a little too long; to bring out the fresher, smoother skin underneath, gentle dermabrasing (sloughing off of the skin) does the trick. To accelerate the natural process of cell regeneration, you need a foaming treatment lotion used with a slightly abrasive applicator. I use my Dermabrase/35 (good for all skins) twice a day, but for average use, once at night is enough to bring about results. Dermabrasing stimulates new cells, improves the skin's texture and helps clear pores.

Beware of liquids labeled *fresheners, toners, exfoliators,* anything that claims to clarify the skin with a simple dab of cotton—they may feel nice, smell nice, but cool tap water is more effective for "freshening" —and it won't parch your skin the way those alcohol-based products can; beware, too, of cleansing grains that are supposed to "roll out" blackheads—that just doesn't happen; and of very abrasive pads that can cause excess redness.

MOISTURIZER

This is a must for all skins. It's not an oil, but is made with oil to simulate natural secretions and seal in the skin's moisture supply. It acts as a barrier between your complexion and the elements: wind, cold, low humidity, all of which can affect even oily skin. A moisturizer should also protect against forming permanent expression lines.

Your product should be invisible to the eye but should leave skin moist to the touch, just as natural oils do. I make two moisturizers, Youth/25 Moisturizing Creme for the traditionally softer skin of the young woman, and Moisture/35 for dry skin that is starting to show its age.

Beware of *heavy cremes* that aren't really absorbed by the skin and that make a mess of any makeup that's applied afterward—the two compete with each other. Save the heavier consistencies for night use.

LUBRICATING CREME

Often called a night creme, this is a rich, emollient creme, of a heavier consistency than a moisturizer. Because of its thickness, it is used at night before bedtime, when not followed with makeup. It shouldn't be visible, and any excess should be tissued off after ten minutes. But it should leave a softening residue on the face.

Beware of *collagen cremes*—that's just a fancy name for another gimmick (and reminiscent of bee jelly's short-lived fame); *hormone creme*—the FDA limits the percentage of hormones a manufacturer can put in its creme, and the amount is so small it couldn't make any sizable difference (and that's still not saying they would do any good in any *topical* dose); *neck creme, eye creme,* etc.—ridiculous! The skin does not have little sensors that shout, "You've left the jawline. Switch to neck creme!" A good creme will bring its softening agents to all areas without discrimination. That's why I recommend my original formulation, Contour/35—it has no restrictions.

NOTE: Lubricating creme is only necessary on dry areas, and then only at night. Dry skin is usually prevalent among women over thirty-five—however, factors such as climate, career and your own chemistry must be considered.

EYE MAKEUP REMOVER (*optional*)

This skin-care product is necessary only if you use a lot of eye makeup and find it difficult to remove at night. Oil-based and water-proof mascaras and eye shadows are particularly resistant to most cleansers. You want a remover that will not tug at the delicate skin of the eye area, yet do an effective job (makeup that isn't completely removed tends to slip into the thin lines under the eyes and deepen them as you sleep). The product should be a light creme that won't smudge or smear makeup or sting or blur the eyes—an important concern of contact-lens wearers. Like my "No-Rub" Gentle/Easy Eye Make-up Remover, it should moisturize the skin as well.

Beware of liquids that have a drying, detergent effect on the eyelids, greasy remover pads that catch lashes and heavy cremes that drag the skin.

SENSIBLE SELECTION

When shopping for skin-care products, be discriminating and use common sense. Describe what you want to the saleswoman, and evaluate her sales pitch carefully. Don't let an eager representative steer you away from your list with her well-rehearsed promises. Ask for a demonstration, and if you are disappointed, bid a quick thank-you before you turn on your heels. Remember the motto of most sales staffs: No obligation to buy. Take that advice when necessary.

After experimenting with an on-counter video system, displaying a short tape describing the treatment line, I found it to be a helpful aid to both the beauty shoppers and the ever-changing saleswomen. My partner, Harry Steinfield, had the idea to develop this system and use it to train Shorell demonstrators and inform customers. It was tested in Canada where we sell to cosmetic boutiques. Today many companies are following suit—try them. (NOTE: skin "toys" on counters that you slide around to try to determine your skin "type" are fun but useless.)

ON CHOOSING PRODUCTS ACCORDING TO . . .

Skin type: This is a very tricky business since most women have a composite complexion—not a "type" at all. But often products are labeled "for dry skin" or "for oily skin." If faced with this kind of choice, opt for the one that suits your predominant skin type. (*Note:* If using an oily-skin-type cleanser on slightly dry areas, use your moisturizer afterward to compensate. Or use two different cleansers—one for oily areas and one for dry. This can be complicated; it requires separate latherings.)

Stay away from these useless products: toners and fresheners marketed for dry skin; astringent lotions for oily skin.

Age range: My own line is divided into two categories, the Youth/25 line and the Contour/35 line, as a guideline to distinguish between young and mature skin. You must consider not only your age but also the visible age of your complexion. If you choose products according to your chronological age only, you can be misled, just as the man who wrote to me saying he achieved the best results from Moisture/35, but thought "mature skin" belonged only to those sixty and older! I explained to him that I know a grandmother in her sixties from Goldsboro, North Carolina, who uses my Youth/25 moisturizing creme —she says that's all her skin needs, despite her age and frequent exposure to the sun and wind (she loves the outdoors!). That lady's skin is undoubtedly moist for her age and probably always was. The point is this: pay attention to your individual needs.

Again, use common sense. If you have very dry skin at an early age or dry patches at any age, use the more concentrated products right away: the heavy creme at night, the gentler formulation of cleanser. If in doubt, take your complexion composite with you when you shop for skin-care products (and makeup, too).

SIXTY COMMON ALLERGENS

Note: The following is a list of cosmetic ingredients known to cause allergic reactions. To avoid even the most minor irritation, none of the products you select should contain any of these. None of the ones I manufacture do.

Acacia
Alizarin
Alkaline earth sulfides
Alum
Aluminum acetate
Aluminum chloride
Aluminum sulphate
Arrowroot
Benzaldehyde
Betanaphthol
Boric acid
Cocoa butter
Cornstarch
Cresol
Dibromofluorescein
Formaldehyde
Geraniol
Gum arabic
Gum karaya
Gum tragacanth
Henna
Lead compounds
Lycopodium
Oil of almond
Oil of bay
Oil of bergamot
Oil of cananga
Oil of cassia
Oil of citronella
Oil of cottonseed

Oil of coriander
Oil of eucalyptus
Oil of heliotropine
Oil of jasmine
Oil of lemon
Oil of linseed
Oil of neroli
Oil of orange
Oil of orris
Oil of spearmint
Oil of wintergreen
Orris root
Oxalic acid
Phenol
Phenoformaldehyde resins
p-Phenylenediamine resins
Quince seed
Resorcinol
Rice starch
Rosin
Salicylic acid
Shellac
Sulfonamide resins
Water soluble aniline dyes
Wheat starch
Wool fat (crude lanolin)
Zinc chloride
Zinc salicylate
Zinc stearate
Zinc sulfate

DO WHAT YOU CAN LIVE WITH MOST COMFORTABLY

Seven minutes—that's the time limit Hal and I imposed on each other to get in and out of the bathroom in the morning so that neither of us would be late for work.

Women who wear light makeup and men (even including shaving) shouldn't need more time than that to get ready in the morning and before getting into bed at night. That's all it takes for a smooth, glowing skin—only a fraction of the time we spend thinking about food. But make it a habit, not the crash-diet type of program you slide on and off.

Here's the plan:

SEVEN MINUTES IN THE MORNING

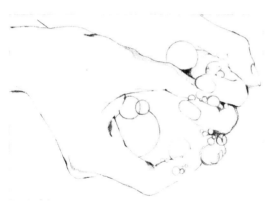

Step One   time: 30 seconds

Wet your hands with warm water. Pour a capful of *liquid cleanser* into your palm. Rub palms together until a lather develops. Rinse hands with slightly hotter water.

Sudsing face.

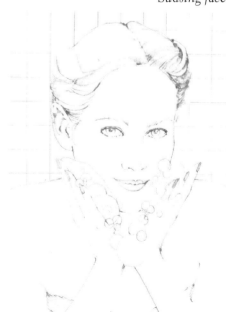

Washing hands.

Step Two   time: 60 seconds

Pour another cupful of cleanser into your palm and make a second lather.

Wash your face and throat with the lather for 30 seconds. Rinse your

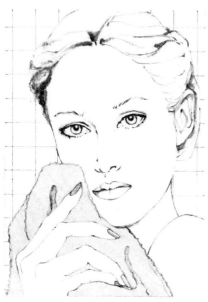

Step Two (continued)

face with warm, then cool water. Pat dry softly with a towel.

Applying moisturizer.

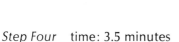

Patting dry.

Step Three time: 2 minutes

With your fingertips, apply *moisturizer* to your face, patting very lightly around the eyes. *Do not rub.* Wait 90 seconds and blot any excess, again taking care not to rub.

Step Four time: 3.5 minutes

A light makeup of mascara, lipstick and, if necessary, blusher.

Optional Step: Dermabrasing

If you're like me and you want to use your dermabrasing liquid and applicator twice a day, make this your third step. For the dermabrasing technique, follow At Night, Step Four. (Moisturizer and makeup then become steps Four and Five respectively.)

Because I apply very little makeup in the morning, I hardly go over my time limit. But if you like more of a look, add an extra five minutes and see Chapter 7 for shortcuts.

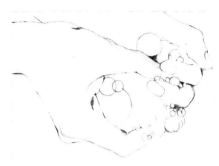

Step One   time: 30 seconds

Wet your hands with warm water. Pour a capful of *liquid cleanser* into your palm. Rub palms together until a lather develops. Rinse hands with slightly hotter water. Dry hands.

Washing hands.

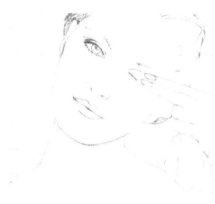

Step Two   time: 60 seconds (if necessary)

Dab a small amount of *eye makeup remover* on a fingertip and gently apply it around a closed eye. As gently, tissue away creme and makeup, always going away from the eye, from the lid to the tips of the lashes, from the inner to the outer corners. Repeat on the other eyelid.

Removing eye makeup.

Step Three   time: 60 seconds

Rinse hands with warm water. Pour a second capful of cleanser into a palm and make a lather. Wash your face and throat for 30 seconds. Rinse your face with warm water. Pat dry softly with a towel.

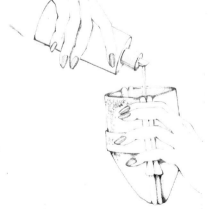

Step Four   time: 3 minutes

Wet your *applicator* with warm water. Pour a capful of your *dermabrasing lotion* into the applicator and squeeze until a lather forms. Using a counterclockwise motion, lightly

Preparing Dermabrase application.

Step Four (*continued*)

go over your face for 1 minute.
Rinse 3 times with warm water.
Using the side of the sponge, go
over your face again for another
minute, concentrating on any oily
areas like the sides of the nose. Go
over the entire face one last time.

Rinse face 3 times with warm
water, then 6 splashes of cold. Dry
with a soft towel.

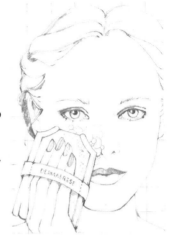

Dermabrasing.

Step Five time: 90 seconds

Repeat the morning *moisturizer*
step, using *lubricating creme* if the
skin is dry or lined. Take special
care around the eyes.

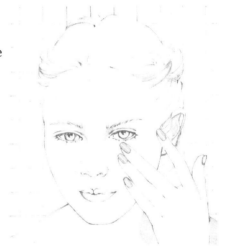

Applying lubricating creme.

Hints in Hindsight

· *On scheduling new habits*: If you're a career woman constantly on the
move, you've probably got your beauty time geared into your schedule.
But if you work at home, you may not be as disciplined—it's easy to
put off washing your face until the kids have left for school—but then
the phone rings, the grocery delivery arrives . . . you never get to *you*.

Set your priorities. Let the breakfast dishes wait. Start establishing a good pattern right away to keep you on the right skin-care track.

- *On hands:* Always start with clean hands. If not, you're just rubbing in dirt and spreading possibly harmful bacteria to products.
- *On removing makeup:* If you forget once or twice, nothing catastrophic will happen, aside from messy bed linens. But neglect is something that easily becomes a habit, a bad habit.
- *On washcloths:* I never use them because they tend to collect bacteria. I don't know who invented them, but I hope he doesn't have any more bright ideas!
- *On dermabrasing:* Once a day is a good practice to follow for fairly tolerant skin. However, once a week can be too much for those with skin that reddens at the mere sight of an abrasive sponge (redheads especially). Be the best judge of your skin's needs (both face and body). Note: If your skin reddened because you were too rough, stop for two days, then start again, with a much gentler hand.
- *On rinsing:* I like to finish with cool to cold water, especially after dermabrasing. It tightens pores, stimulates skin.
- *On patting dry:* Use a clean face towel every day.
- *On at-home facials:* I'm not crazy about any kind of facial that calls for a lot of dabbing on of cremes. You might, however, steam your face occasionally by holding it over a pot of just-boiled water, with a towel draped over your head. Do this after cleansing, before dermabrasing.

If you like the idea of having the kind of beauty pampering you'd get at an expensive salon or spa, my Seven-Day at Home Beauty Plan is for you. It combines the basics of skin care (for face and body) with beauty chores (shaving, shampooing . . .) in a way that combines work with pleasure—such as my treatment bath.

The best part of this at-home plan is that you can make every week like a week at a spa. If you're on vacation, devote seven full days to fitness (add low-cal gourmet menus every day, along with a couple of exercise classes, a daily jog, maybe even have a professional masseuse visit in your own bedroom). When you're doing your nine-to-five, the following schedule can be adapted to suit your personal timetable— without sacrificing any of the terrific results. You can even start slowly, adding one or two days' worth of treats each week. But I think you'll like this beneficial pampering so much you'll want to plunge right in.

Note: All body-care steps (manicure, treatment bath, etc.) are detailed in Chapter 4, *Your Home Beauty Spa.*

MY SEVEN DAY AT HOME BEAUTY PLAN

SATURDAY

MORNING

Start your weekend off right: sleep as late as you need to and see your complexion in its optimum form. But once you're awake, don't lounge around. Get up and start your blood moving right away—or else you may never get going!

Cleanse your face as you usually do, but after patting dry, don't apply anything. Wait 1 hour (have breakfast) before you start your new skin-care plan.

AFTERNOON

Evaluating session: Examine your complexion as described in Chapter 3.

Determine what products you need, those you can do without.

Decide to spend the next couple of hours doing a little beauty shopping.

EVENING

Start your P.M. skin care ritual tonight, even (especially) if you were out very late.

If you scrutinized your products carefully before buying, they should be familiar to you. Remember my first skin-care resolution!

Promise never to go to sleep without removing your makeup and cleansing your face thoroughly.

SUNDAY

Your A.M. skin care ritual begins today, and there's no better beginning for your day of rest.

Treat yourself to a "spa" brunch: an attractively prepared, low-cal, high-nutrition meal —a cold seafood platter of mussels, shrimp and clams, tomato and red onion salad, fresh raspberries and a 3-ounce glass of champagne. Lavish for one, divine for two!

After an exciting day, start thinking about the week ahead and give yourself the spa-grooming treatment from head to toe: take a long bath, de-fuzz and condition legs, add a little sparkle to your hands and feet with a mani/pedicure.

Enjoy dinner wrapped in a luxurious robe: at-home elegance.

Your P.M. skin care (don't forget to dermabrase).

MONDAY

Your A.M. skin care.

Mid-afternoon skin-relief break: if your skin is showing the stress of Monday-back-to-work-blues any day of the week, give your face a mini-cleanse. Without removing your eye makeup, wash and moisturize.

Reapply blush and a little lipstick. You'll have more energy than a midday candy bar can give!

Think about investing in a hand-held shower unit with steam feature to give yourself a wonderful skin treatment (skin loves humidity).

Your P.M. skin care before bed.

TUESDAY	WEDNESDAY	THURSDAY	FRIDAY

Your A.M. skin care.

Your A.M. skin care. If your skin will tolerate it, dermabrase in the morning, too, from now on. But go lightly: start with only 1 minute for the first few days.

Your A.M. skin care.

Your A.M. skin care.

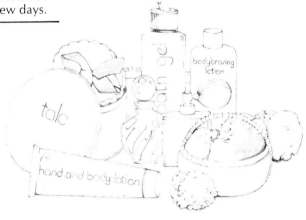

Invest in yourself: join a gym or yoga class near your office. Attend 3 or more times a week. Pick up a fast, healthful lunch on your way back: try yogurt and fresh nuts and raisins.

Mid-afternoon skin relief break, if needed.

Mid-afternoon skin-relief break, if needed.

Mid-afternoon skin-relief break, if needed.

Mid-afternoon skin relief break, if needed.

If you usually take showers (or even if you don't), tonight indulge in my treatment bath: a long, nourishing soak (for the skin and the psyche!), followed with body lotion, a pat of talc, a splash of fragrance.

Your P.M. skin care. (If bathing right before bed, cleanse your face first.)

Your P.M. skin care.

Mini-spa touch-up: Take 30 minutes to fix any chips in your nail polish, to take a few strokes of the razor under arms, to shampoo hair (maybe you'll start with a 20-minute conditioning pack, rinse and wash before using polish).

Your P.M. skin care.

Before an important date, try my instant-acting face mask. It's actually a light foam that smoothes into the skin, gives an instant lift. Just cleanse, apply mask, and sponge off after 3 minutes with warm water. Then moisturizer, makeup—and sparkle!

Your P.M. skin care.

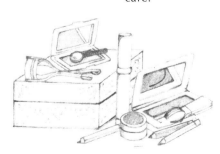

CHAPTER 4

Your Home Beauty Spa

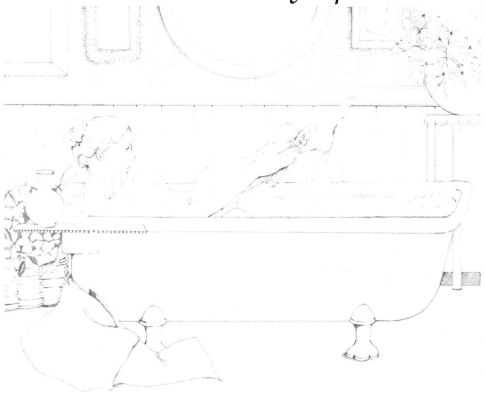

Y<small>OUR</small> complexion doesn't stop at your neck, but softness can, if you're not careful. I realized that soon after I began devoting much of my time to skin care. It always seemed as though I could use a few extra hours just to care for all a woman's grooming needs. But rather than admit defeat, I tried a little organization: instead of scrambling for ten minutes here to shampoo, fifteen minutes there for a manicure, I put together an extensive beauty shape-up program of one solid hour. I lock myself in my beauty haven (the john, but well-equipped to meet all my needs) and get down to my beautifying work: a bath or a shower, shampooing, de-fuzzing, a manicure and pedicure and all the little extras (talc, fragrance) that turn clean into . . . memorable.

GOOD-HEALTH CHECKS

Because beauty is impossible without good health, and because good health is so much more important than good looks, every woman should consider having these good-health checks periodically (once a year is the general rule, especially if you're over thirty-five) to prevent problems. If you visit your gynecologist or family doctor yearly, she or he can perform almost all of these in short order.

1. *High blood-pressure check*. This leading cause of heart disease affects nearly 8 percent of all women. Visit one of the free mobile units if you can't get to your doctor.

2. *Cancer checks*. Cancer can be stayed if discovered early enough.
   - Breast cancer: supplement your doctor's check with your own monthly exam at home, after each period. Ask her/him to show you how.
   - Cervical cancer: a simple Pap smear should always be a part of your yearly check-up.
   - Cancer of the colon: this check is especially important for women over forty.

3. *Blood checks for anemia and diabetes*. Both these ills appear more frequently in women than men and should be part of the tests run routinely on your blood.

4. *Urinalysis* is another routine check that measures blood sugar, important in the diagnosis of diabetes and of bladder infections, which have become very common of late.

5. *Glaucoma check*. 20/20 vision doesn't make you immune to eye disease or a future loss of vision. A full eye exam, thirty to sixty minutes long, is a must every two or three years. The glaucoma check takes only a couple of minutes; other checks are for vision and for side vision, focusing, reflexes, perception and the proper prescription for glasses or contact lenses.

The time you spend on these checks is the most valuable of all your beauty time. Don't stint.

From <u>Bath</u>room to Beauty Room

The ultimate bath has a luxuriously appointed tub and counters and drawers for all your beauty equipment: lotions, makeups, hair tools, perfume bottles, towels, robes—it's a dressing room-cum-bath. But realistically, most of us must work with far less lavish space and equipment.

You can, however, still have a beauty haven to call your own. First, organize your space as best you can between the medicine chest and the vanity of your basin. Group together items for: skin care, makeup, manicure, body care, shaving, etc. Have all your beauty items in the bathroom, even if you must store extra towels in a closet and keep in the bathroom only those you'll use at any one time.

Second, beautify the john. A velvety towel, fluffed from careful laundering, always adds elegance. Have your bath towel or sheet folded within easy reach. (If you've been reminding yourself for months to buy new towels, make your next after-work shopping night the time to get a matched set—towel, bath sheet, mat—in a color you love. You needn't wallpaper to rid the room of clinical characteristics: two coats of a soft color over a dingy white or gray will add style. But don't go too dark—even a bright red will diffuse your light. Peach, beige, pale lemon, light mushroom are possibilities. If you like the clean appeal of white, choose a bright, crisp gloss. If you're creative, stencil a small design around the room at eye level for interest. A mirrored wall opposite a mirrored medicine chest gives you a total field of vision; fluorescent tubing gives you a clear view when sunlight (the best light) isn't available. Most women never think of putting flowers in the bathroom, but why not? You'll be inspired by their beauty and fragrance. Plants that love humidity and need a minimum of light will thrive in even a windowless bathroom. Dried flowers and greens can be scented with an atomizer of your favorite cologne. Don't save candles for those rare nights when you soak to music in a scented tub; use them—unlit— as a permanent part of your decor.

When your bathroom is the size of a closet, as are most of those in newer apartment buildings, use space as efficiently as possible. Don't try to put up shelves if space is so tight that too vigorous toweling would topple the works. Too much decorating may get in your way: use prints or pictures (framed to avoid their being warped from the humidity) instead of plants. Keep as much as you can off the limited counter space so that you'll have the room to lay out specific tools as you need them.

Always make the time to retreat to your beauty room—and make it clear to all that this time is yours alone. Have a special gown or robe to slip into when you've finished your ministrations, to prolong the luxurious feeling that comes from turning good grooming into all-out pampering.

Water Therapies

While not as complex as your facial needs, the body's complexion does often have its imperfections: dry, flaky skin of the limbs and joints (elbows, knees, ankles); oily chest and back; "bumps" on the hips, thighs and buttocks; sensitive skin anywhere. To improve your body skin, you must care for it with the same five principles of complexion care.

By now, most should be a part of your conscious daily life: eating well, staying out of the sun. But direct action will have wonderful results. That's why showers and baths should be carefully thought out— these "water therapies" *work!*

Just as you selected the right products for your complexion care, do so for your body. But remember—just as you had to pick and choose your way through a myriad of skin preparations, you will have to do the same when gearing up for the tub.

POTIONS AND LOTIONS

The list of bath products available goes on and on, partially because these are packaged as gift items. Your husband probably won't present you with a jar of moisturizer on Valentine's Day, but he might very well get you a fancy bottle of bath salts. By the way, if he does, take it back. (I'll tell you why soon.) The truth is, the right products are much too important to be chosen for you. (Tactfully tell your spouse or beau not to be tempted by pretty packaging—bows and ribbons look just as nice on boxes from Tiffany's or a box of long-stemmed roses!) Examine the skin on each area of your body and acquire what you need from the following bathing bounty.

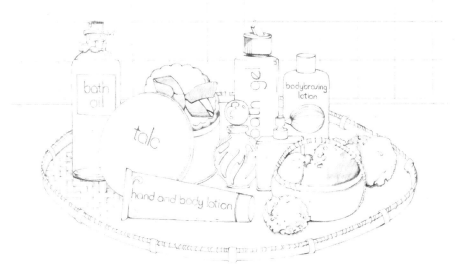

BATH GEL

This is the product I find myself using most frequently. It should be a moisturizing as well as a cleansing product, to be added as the bath water runs (or used with an applicator in the shower). Optimally, it should be lightly bubbling and nicely scented though not if your skin is the slightest bit sensitive. The innermost skin of the genitals can be sensitive to the *slightest* ingredient, even when your arms and legs show no reaction. In fact, urinary-tract infections can be caused or aggravated by fragranced products. (If you experience any such tendencies, you will probably be more comfortable taking showers than baths.)

We are so used to thinking we have to see soapsuds to really get clean that we often think a bath gel isn't enough. But in truth, it is. Use a sponge to soak up the light sudsy bubbles and then use it to wash your skin—this gentle stimulation is good for circulation. If your gel moisturizes as does my Bath Formula Gelée, your skin will rinse clean and smooth, but not taut.

Beware of bubbling bath salts and *crystals*—these don't accomplish anything except to increase dryness; also of *bath milks*—if I thought milk did any good, I'd go straight to the supermarket, buy two gallons, pour it into the tub and jump in!

BATH OIL

A treatment product to soothe dry, itchy skin, bath oil is for the woman who is sensitive to fabrics like wool, stiff cottons, and even synthetics, which may cause discomfort, itching, and often, rashes. You want one that cleanses as well, thereby eliminating the need for soap, another possible irritant to tender skin. The cleansing action should be discernibly effective, without any need for vigorous scrubbing. Like my Body Treatment 35/Bath Oil, it should shield the skin from irritation as it cleanses as well as lubricate, soothe, and be completely fragrance-free. The treatment product you select should leave skin so soft you won't even need to apply any after-bath cremes or lotions (until, possibly, the next morning) And a relaxing twenty-minute bath needn't be taboo anymore for anyone with sensitive skin.

Beware of bath oils that are *greasy*—they coat the skin surface, leaving it slick to the touch, and without necessarily helping the skin retain moisture; moisture retention is the true secret of combating the irritated-skin syndrome. *Perfumed oils* must also be ruled out, as fragrance has been proved to be a major allergen for many people.

BODYBRASING LOTION

"Bodybrasing" is as important and as beautifying a step for the body as dermabrasing is for the complexion. Too often, that top layer of dead skin cells hangs around a bit too long, especially after a suntan or burn or great deal of exposure to the elements. Elbows, heels, knees get the worst of it, but no part of the body is immune. Gentle body-brasing gradually smoothes out those tiny bumps that make skin rough in areas like the backs of the thighs and the arms and the sides of the hips. The proper lotion and applicator should elminate these woes, unclog pores and revitalize sun-damaged skin, too.

Because body skin is much tougher than that of the face, you want a strong working lotion that is used with a fairly abrasive pad or a natural sponge, like a loofah. My Bodybrase/35 comes with its own applicator.

Beware of clarifying systems that claim they will remove cellulite or fat pockets. Exercise alone can do that. And they may not even do the job you should expect them to do. Clarifying liquids that work like alcohol-based astringents or that contain fragrance that is part alcohol, can irritate rather than smoothe. Always refer back to the list of known and suspected irritants before investing in any skin-care products (See page 00).

NOTE: Always follow the directions of the specific product you are using, taking special care to follow directions on frequency of use and the amount of pressure you exert.

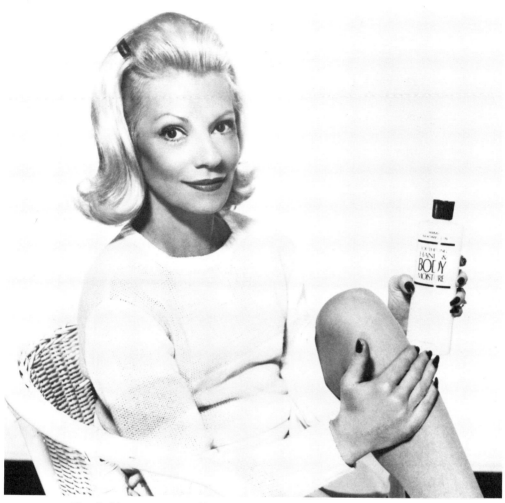

Good skin care means all-over skin care—for head-to-toe smoothness and glow.

BODY LOTION

We don't notice it as readily, but the body is just as subject to moisture loss as the face. Like a facial moisturizer, a body lotion must nourish and protect the skin's suppleness. This is especially important for those with very dry, flaky skin; used after a bath-oil treatment, the lotion doubles the buffer effect.

The lotion you use must be rich and creamy and should leave a thin shield on the skin surface to help retain its moisture; it should be effective, too, on your hands and your feet. It can be fragranced, to match your perfume if you like, or fragrance-free if that's what you prefer or if your skin is sensitive or allergy-prone. That's why I developed twin lotions: my Youthening Hand and Body Moisture is made both with fragrance and without.

Beware of accumulating a multitude of cremes: hand lotion, foot lubricant, elbow *grease!* The theory that the heavier the lubricant, the more it can soften, is not accurate. No creme will penetrate the toughened, callused skin so often found on heels and knees. You must get rid of calluses, of rough patches at elbows, ankles, anywhere, through mild bodybrasing, which removes the built-up layers of old skin cells; then lubricate with your *one* lotion.

SPONGES

A bath sponge is great for getting the skin's circulation up and for thorough cleansing, too. There is a great variety available—from the inexpensive dime-store kind to those costing over a hundred dollars— hard as that is to believe! Here are some choices:

- a rounded natural sponge
- a loofah sponge (the kind that reminds you of a giant piece of shredded wheat, but softens in your bath water)
- a sponge mitt that fits over your hand like a glove
- a soft-bristle brush—the kind with an extra-long handle is wonderful for reaching every inch of your back.

You can treat yourself to a wardrobe of sponges, but have at least one that really soaks up the water in the tub, as well as your oil or gel for the shower (you'll find you need less of these because a sponge remains sudsy for quite a long time).

TALC

I love the satiny-smooth finish talc gives, whether it's pure baby powder sprinkled straight from its own perforated container or lavishly pressed from a large puff that sits in a special holder.

Scented powder to match your fragrance is a wonderful luxury, but I think you'll find the unscented, plain white variety satisfactory for absorbing surface moisture that can cause uncomfortable friction (moisture often missed by your towel).

PERFUME: YOUR UNSPOKEN MESSAGE

Fragrance, though not a bath product, has wonderful, long-lasting effects when used afterward. Your scent can become your signature, a special part of you, and should be carefully chosen to suit your personality and to please your taste. Perfume is a terrific treat, as I found while developing my own fragrance, and should never be overlooked—its powers are potent yet always mysterious.

Selecting a perfume isn't always easy, but it's an interesting task—and a rewarding one too. Here are some ideas:

· Always test a perfume on yourself. No matter how great it smells on someone else, it will be different on you (each of us has a unique chemistry that will cause varying reactions when combined with the chemistry of the fragrance).

· Try no more than two perfumes at any one time, one on each wrist, to make an accurate determination. Compare the scents at 10-minute intervals. First the top notes emerge, then the middle notes, finally the base notes, altering the scent each time. Because the base notes last the longest, you should like these the best.

· Solve the perfume vs. cologne debate by evaluating your skin: thin, dry skin reacts best to the oil-based *perfume* concentration; skin that is oily, especially on the chest and back, might be more comfortable with lighter concentrations of *cologne* or *eau de toilette*. The oils in perfume help dry skin retain the fragrance. Oily skin doesn't have the problem of vanishing fragrance and doesn't need these extra oils, unless you want the stronger scent.

Other choices:

creme sachets: These come in pretty compacts, easy to slip in your purse, to dab on discreetly anywhere.

atomizers: Filled with your preferred concentration, these diffuse the spray for easy misting on clothes, the alternate way of wearing scent for those with sensitive or allergic skin. Mist hair, too.

perfumed talc and body lotions: Use these to layer on your fragrance, one of the most luxurious feelings there is.

· Be creative with your fragrance. Saturate cotton balls and tuck into purses and pockets when dry to create a scented aura; for an extra-refreshing cooldown in summer, chill cologne in the refrigerator; mist fragrance on dried flowers and leaves around your home and office.

· Remember that, though your sense of smell is among the most discriminating of the senses, it can get used to your favorite scent —that's why it is possible for companies to launch new fragrances all the time. To reawaken your awareness, switch to another scent for a few weeks (invest in a small size) and then go back to your perfume with renewed enthusiasm.

THE BODYBRASING SHOWER

for · a refreshing morning wake-up
· an after-sport polish
· an après-sun cooldown
· renewal of sunburned skin

1. Cleanse face, patting off excess moisture.

2. Step into the shower and saturate your body with water. If shampooing, let water run through your hair.

3. Lather hair, massage scalp. If you're using a dandruff shampoo, leave it in for a while before rinsing. If a regular shampoo, you can rinse now.

4. Cleanse body with gel or oil applied to your sponge. Squeeze the sponge to get a lather and slather it all over, adding water to the sponge to reactivate the product as you need it.

THE BODYBRASING BATH

for · a revitalizing ritual after a long day
· before a special evening
· a rejuvenating treatment the morning after a night on the town

1. Add bath oil or gel to running water.

2. Cleanse face as the tub fills.

3. Apply moisturizer or creme liberally, then slip into the tub and soak.

4. Gently use sponge to help the cleansing action of your bath product, sopping up the treated water and squeezing the sponge over shoulders, back, everywhere.

5. Now it's time to bodybrase. Wet the applicator thoroughly. Now pour in two capfuls of your treatment lotion and squeeze until a foam appears.

6. Gently go over your back, your elbows and your knees for about 1 minute or until skin is slightly rosy, not *red*. Next use on dry or bumpy areas like the thighs, the hips, the upper arms, the shoulders if needed. Always go over the skin with a light hand in a counterclockwise motion—never rub back and forth. Don't be harsh: those bumps won't go away in one session. A little each day for the first few days and then every other day is usually enough. Rinse and use on heels and ankles, rinsing one foot before going to the other to avoid slipping.

If you're in the shower, move slightly out of the water stream as you go over each area to avoid washing away the foam too soon.

If you are in the tub, try to keep area you are bodybrasing out of the water as much as possible for most effective results.

7. In the shower, rinse off thoroughly, first with warm, then cool,

(continued on page 70)

water. Bathers might like a quick spritz under the shower as a final rinse.

Note: if you are going to de-fuzz, do it now and then finish with the following steps. (For shaving tips, see page 71.)

8. Before drying completely, shake off excess water and generously apply body lotion. Let it soak into your skin. Apply your moisturizer/creme to work along with this.

9. Use a towel to polish or buff your skin: this will blot up any unabsorbed lotion. Now blot any moisturizer/creme.

10. Powder at your pulse points, and around any folds of skin that might irritate each other: under the arms, between the legs, under each breast. If you use deodorant or its stronger form, anti-perspirant, apply it now.

11. Apply your fragrance if you wish, *as you wish*.

SHOWER BONUS	TUB BONUS
To turn your shower into a real steam room, treat yourself to a steam attachment. The device delivers a steady warm mist with either the hand-held model (for greatest control) or the wall attachment that frees you for other duties.	To make your soak most enjoyable, get a tray that bridges the width of the tub or attaches to the open side. It will hold your sponge and other beauty tools, as well as a book or magazine to read when you're just plain relaxing.

Beauty Methods

Your at-home spa isn't just for cleansing; it's for beautifying, too. That can mean adding the sparkle of polish to your nails and toes, or the more prosaic de-fuzzing process. Whatever beauty method is next on your list, there are ways of making it less taxing and the results longer lasting—and that translates to a better-looking you.

HAIR TODAY, GONE TODAY

The best thing to do with unwanted hair is to get rid of it. But finding a quick and effective means of doing just that isn't so easy.

Today, with all the chemical agents flooding the market, the preferred method is still the safety razor with a cartridge-type blade—nothing dangerous to handle, inexpensive enough and speedy to use.

TAKE IT OFF, TAKE IT ALL OFF WITH . . .	TO HAVE HANDY
· a scented liquid soap lathered with an ivory-handled brush *or* · your favorite cleanser *or* · a shaving foam (regular only; menthol can irritate) *and* your razor!	a mirror for checking the backs of legs, upper arms, etc.

I've found the best way to shave is in the evening, just after a bath or shower. The hairs have been softened by the water and come off quite easily. After the bath, let the water run out of the tub and sit on the edge of the tub, a towel under you to avoid slipping, legs facing in.

1. Turn on the faucet and wet your legs thoroughly (if you haven't just left the tub or shower). Water opens pores for a closer shave.

2. Lather up generously, but not too thickly, or your first strokes will be all foam, no hair.

3. Use single, long strokes in the direction opposite that of your natural hair growth for the cleanest shave. Rinse the razor completely each time. Continue until you've removed hair and foam all the way around your calves.

4. Rinse legs completely and use a mirror to check for stray hairs. Remove any hairs you might have missed, after applying just a bit of lather on these areas. (Never shave *dry*.) Rinse again.

5. Adapt your technique to the area you're shaving. For the thighs, stand up in the shower, bending over slightly to rinse the razor under running water. For the often difficult area around the knees, first try angling your razor around the bent knee as you sit; if you're not completely successful, try standing. When shaving under the arms, or the arms themselves, try standing at the sink in front of a wall mirror. Always change the direction of your strokes so that it opposes the direction of hair growth, especially under the arms.

6. Rinse well, ending with cool to cold water to close pores.

7. Use body lotion and buff as you would after a bath or shower.

NOTES:
Never shave dry legs/arms/anywhere. Always wet and lather.

ALTERNATIVES TO THE SAFETY RAZOR

The electric razor. There are many women who prefer this method as it eliminates the nick factor. However, a large number of people who use it do develop razor burn afterward. To eliminate this, use either a preshave product or a liberal sprinkling of baby powder on the area to be shaved: this draws up any moisture that might hamper the smooth flow of the razor's numerous tiny blades. Always shave before bath/shower when using this method. A good follow-up cleansing will help prevent irritation. Always clean the razor after use with the wire brush included with the set, or with a pipe cleaner.

Depilatories. Available in lotion or foam, the products are applied and left in place to dissolve the hairs, then rinsed away. The regrowth process is somewhat delayed, but there are two drawbacks. First, many women are allergic or sensitive to certain chemical ingredients they contain; and you have to buy the product before you can test it. Second, the odor is often unpleasant; depending on your olfactory sense, you may or may not be able to tolerate it.

Waxing. This is the most lasting of the temporary hair-removal methods but you need great willpower to perform the technique on yourself—or sufficient pocket money to have it professionally done. Most at-home kits direct you to melt the wax, paint it on and pull it off when hard. At many salons, a newer method is available: a soft, liquid wax is applied and removed right away with strips of fabric—this causes less pain. I don't think you ever get used to the sensation, but many women swear by waxing, right up to their bikini lines! It's tolerated so well (by men, too) because it need only be done once every two or three months, depending on how fast your body hair grows back.

Electrolysis. This is the most time- and money-consuming method, but unwanted hair is permanently removed. What actually happens is this: the root of each individual hair is destroyed by a tiny bit of electric current, one hair at a time; this is a lengthy process where the legs are concerned. Most women opt for this method for removal of facial hair (a hairline above the upper lip for instance), as the area is not too great.

There is some pain involved and only limited areas can be worked on at a time—you couldn't take more! As with any de-fuzzing method, this one has its drawbacks, but for many, the fact that the hair is permanently removed makes this a sound choice. (Yes, women have had their entire legs done.)

Note: In rare instances, some hairs may grow back.

Never shave before going out into the sun; skin will be too sensitive and subject to burning.

Always try to shave at night, to give skin a chance to rest, especially under the arms, as applying deodorant immediately after shaving can cause irritation. Apply deodorant the next morning.

A PERFECT TEN

A very small percentage of women have naturally lovely nails; the rest of us have to spend a good deal of time not only manicuring, but guarding against chips, splits, lost nails. It's no wonder few of us want to take that needed time to beautify our nails. But this is no place to scrimp on good looks—our hands play too important a part to let go unattended. A weekly manicure (and pedicure) by a beautician or by you yourself is a must. If your schedule is limited, omit colored polish, the real time-consumer; finish with a clear gloss—it looks very pretty and you won't have to worry about the color clashing with any last-minute changes in your wardrobe.

Before You Start

· Check the weather report. On a damp, rainy evening, your polish will never dry! Put off your manicure, if you are using polish, until the clouds break.
· Allow plenty of time, especially if you are using polish. Applying polish isn't a good thing to squeeze in between other chores.
· If you're going to give yourself a pedicure, do it before you do your hands. In fact, do everything before you do your hands: brush your your teeth, wash your face . . . so that your manicured nails won't have to come into contact with water again till the next morning.
· Certainly, if you're going to bathe or shower, do so before starting on your nails. The water is excellent for softening cuticles.

Exception: remove old polish before getting wet and take care of step #2, below, in the tub.

NOTE: Unless indicated, the following steps can be applied to a manicure and a pedicure both. Always do the pedicure first, if you're doing both.

The Manicure/Pedicure

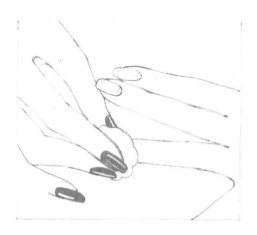

1. *Thoroughly remove all your old polish.* Use a bit of cotton around an orangewood stick to clean around the cuticles. Go over each nail once more with a clean piece of cotton and remover. Rinse hands to wash away traces of the remover.

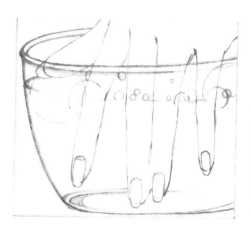

2. *Soak your hands in warm, soapy water.* (Using your cleanser is fine; so is water treated with bath gel/oil.) Scrub carefully under and over nails. Use an orangewood stick to remove any stubborn dirt under or around nails. Rinse in clear water and dry hands completely.

3. *Buff your nails.* Use the creme or powder in a buff kit to massage the nails. The kit should also include a fabric-covered brush for buffing (not one with bristles); this action stimulates circulation, gives nails a rosy glow and smoothes the nail surface for easy polish application.

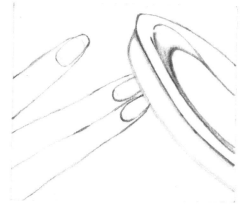

4. *File your nails. Do not cut cuticles.* Use an emery board (the light-colored side) or a metal nail file to even the curve of your nails. Exaggerated shapes such as fine points or square clips often look too unnatural to be attractive and draw too much attention to your hands. Your hands should look well groomed, not made up. Slightly rounded corners, straight sides for support and an easy curve to the edge give the most pleasing shape.

Please do nothing more to your cuticles than keep them clean. If you leave them alone, they will hardly be noticeable. If your

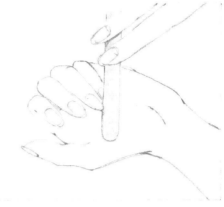

manicurist wants to clip the cuticles, find yourself a new salon.

For the toenails: Clip each nail straight across in a blunt shape, filing only any uneven edges. You'll get a neater finish by using the clippers than by using only a file.

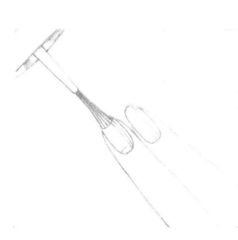

5. *Apply a clear gloss polish* to use alone or as an undercoat to keep color pigments of bright enamels from permeating the nails. I use this same colorless polish as a top coat—no need for a separate finish when one bottle will do both jobs. NOTE: Buy only the polish you need for immediate use. Polish and enamels get thick as they age and using thinners is a pain in the neck (the thin neck of the bottle!).

6. *Use nail enamel if you wish.* Apply color to each nail in three strokes: first stroke on the far right; then a stroke on the far left; then the last, straight down the center. This method assures color on the sides from the start: no more dabbing in the corners after the center of the nail has been done— a surefire way to smudge a smooth coat.

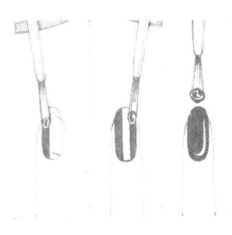

For the toenails: Separate toes with cotton balls or weave a strip of toilet tissue through each to prevent their touching while polish dries. You can start your *mani*cure at this point, but remove the cotton before polishing your fingernails.

Note on color selection: Don't let your choice be dictated by what color is "in." Choose a shade that complements your skin tone. Don't go too light if you have pale skin, or too dark if you have dark skin. Do use matching or complimentary shades of lipstick and polish. And if your nail enamel is suited to lip color that's natural (not *shocking* pink or *flaming* orange or *purplish* blue), you won't have to worry about clashes with clothing.

7. *Allow more than enough time for polish to dry.* The secret is to allow each coat to dry before applying the next. But that's tricky to judge: enamel that looks, even feels, dry to a light touch can still get smudged. Allow five minutes for the gloss undercoat to dry before applying enamel. Wait thirty minutes before applying the second enamel coat, and an hour before applying the final coat of gloss.

Short of knocking yourself out, there's no easy way to pass the time. I try planning my manicure so that polish goes on at the start of a two-hour movie—an interesting one, if I can find it, to ensure that I'm not easily distracted. By the time it's over, my last coat of clear polish has dried and then it's off to sleep.

ON FAKE NAILS

Artificial nail tips are valuable if one nail breaks and ruins the long, lush look of the other nine. But it is too expensive a practice for all ten nails, unless you rarely use your hands or have a live-in expert to replace any tips that fall off during the course of the day. It's not too difficult to guard against losing one tip, but all ten . . . I can't imagine it.

Maintenance is the chief drawback. A nail tip requires that your own nail be filed in a somewhat unnatural shape before the tip is applied; in the case of a loss, you wouldn't want your nail running around "naked" until it fully grows in—you'll want to stay in close proximity to your nail salon. I've lost a tip at the supermarket, at the theater—it can happen anywhere. You might rap your nails against a railing or counter; it's easy to hit the tip in a way that will unhinge it.

But I do not advocate the alternative—the fake nail that is painted and bonded onto your own nails. The real nail is literally suffocated by the artificial material, and that can be harmful. It's far better to have perfectly groomed nails that are on the short side. Use only clear gloss as polish for short nails; colored enamels attract attention, make nails look stubby.

Remember, too, that for many women long, perfectly polished fingernails are not practical. Guitarists, potters and other hobbyists, crackerjack typists, busy mothers will want to keep their necessarily short nails clean and buffed, and perhaps polished with a clear lacquer. Busy hands that proclaim that their owners work and create are beautiful in their own right.

Nail Savers/Time Savers

· Don't be spontaneous about opening packages. Take the time to get a pair of scissors or use the jagged edge of a key.
· Always use a pencil when dialing the telephone, regular or push button.
· Don't untie knots in laces or strings with long nails or tips. Ask someone to help you.
· I love gelatin desserts and can fill up on a bowlful, but in all the time I've eaten it, I've never noticed a positive effect on my nails. Don't indulge for that reason.
· Renew the shine of your manicure with a mid-week coat of gloss. Use enamel only when chips become obvious.
· Use canvas-lined rubber gloves when working in the garden or around the house. They protect the softness of your hands and increase the life of your polish. Even better if you can find them: the disposable plastic gloves that doctors use; they are thinner and afford more dexterity.
· Never apply perfume with polished fingers—ingredients can mar the shiny enamel finish. Use an atomizer.

Relaxation Therapies

Nothing will age a woman's whole being faster than the look of frown lines spanning the forehead, a clenched jaw and a mouth that perpetually pouts. The grimaces, quite unfortunately, are more involuntary than we think. They are often reflex actions to all the stress and tension we store throughout the day—from hassles at work, pressure from the kids,

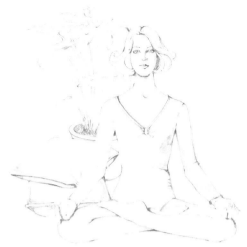

even the dilemma of what to cook for dinner. Everything seems to creep up on us from time to time, almost always all at once.

The real problem with tension is not knowing how to relieve it. Left unchecked, the frown lines deepen, the headaches become more frequent, life is just a bowl of cherry pits.

The solution is simple. Relax. Exhale the tension. There are many ways to accomplish this. All you need to do is choose one. The therapy you want will depend on the tension quota of your average day: lots of stress and strain demands serious techniques.

Sleep is a natural, the universal cure. As soon as you fall asleep, the body eases: the temperature and blood pressure lower, the pulse and breathing rates slow. The body relaxes itself. But falling asleep is often the hardest part. Two updated versions of tried-and-true remedies: a glass of warm milk—add cinnamon and a dash of vanilla if you like; or a cup of tea—not the usual tea, containing caffeine, but a restful herbal such as a camomile or linden tea. A warm bath before bed works wonders, too.

Of course, you can't lie down at the office whenever you're tense. But you can take off your shoes for a few minutes during your lunch hour instead of running out to lunch or to shop. Concentrate on the idea of peacefulness, picture yourself lying on a beach, at the water's edge.

At home, the answer is a midday nap, a custom we should have adopted from our Mediterranean neighbors long ago. Research has shown that your body functions at peak capacity after a short, twenty-minute nap. Try it after lunch, before the kids come home from school, and always on the weekends to help rejuvenate yourself for the week ahead.

NOTE: Studies have proven that Americans who sleep a full seven to eight hours every night live longer!

Yoga is an excellent therapeutic because as it teaches basic meditation, it provides exercise postures that improve flexibility and stature. Fundamentally, you quickly learn to breathe deeply and correctly, inhaling oxygen, which the yogis think of as "energy," exhaling tension. Try a yoga class twice a week at a gym or through private instruction ($7 to $10 a class).

To get you started:

1. Basic yoga breathing. Lie down and spread your fingers across your stomach. Inhale through your nose, pushing out your belly to permit your lungs and diaphragm to fill with air. At first you may really have to push the air down because we are all so very used to sucking in our stomachs to inhale—just the opposite of correct breathing.

Hold the breath for a few seconds. Then with great control, slowly exhale through the mouth, feeling the stomach cavity hollow. Repeat four times and continue breathing this way throughout the next steps.

2. Tension release #1. Still lying flat, bend your right knee against your chest without straining. The left knee is bent, foot flat on the floor. Slowly rotate your right ankle in small circles, starting to the right. Repeat this for a total of four times, then reverse the direction and repeat four more times.

Lower your right foot to the floor, knee bent. Repeat the exercise with your left foot.

3. Tension release #2. Sit up with your legs folded. To ease tension in the neck, drop your head to the right shoulder, but do not move the shoulder—only the head moves. Now bring chin to chest, then bring your head around to the left shoulder, then all the way back and around to the right shoulder again. Do this in one continuous motion. When you've circled around four times, change directions and repeat four times.

4. Lying down flat again, concentrate on your breathing once more. Though you should have been doing this throughout the last two steps, focus on it fully now. To release the tension everywhere in your body, you're going to start by tensing every muscle on the inhale and releasing at once on the exhale. Do this three times.

Now inhale and concentrate on the toes. As you exhale, release all tension from the toes. In your mind, move your attention to your feet and repeat the inhale, exhaling to release any tension in your feet. In the following order, let your mind's eye go over each part of the body, inhaling and exhaling to release any stored tension: ankles, calves, knees, thighs, hips, buttocks, stomach, back, hands, arms, shoulders, neck and head.

Continue this yoga breathing even when all the tension is gone. Imagine yourself as just another star in space, nowhere to go, nothing to do. Remain relaxed, your mind empty, your yoga breathing second nature now, for a full three minutes.

Now slowly sit up and feel yourself refreshed.

Massage is often thought of as a luxury, but those who indulge regularly insist it is a necessity, a part of their weekly routine. Massage relieves the tension that is often stored in our very muscles, that builds up over a period of time—the result of a hectic lifestyle, yet a lifestyle that doesn't include regular exercise. This isn't to say that massage will remedy the effects of lack of exercise—only exercise can do that. But it will go a long way toward alleviating tension.

Be aware of your body's needs. Everyone stores tension in different areas; these will require extra attention by the masseuse. As you get used to massage, you'll learn to work with the various techniques for optimum benefit.

Where to get a massage? You needn't be on a luxury vacation or at a costly spa to avail yourself of one. Most gyms offer the services of a masseuse, as do many beauty salons, particularly those in specialty stores. Many reputable masseuses will visit you at your convenience at home, in the evening or even during a weekend of pampering.

Why have a massage? It's one of the nicer things you can do for yourself, physically and emotionally. And because a lubricating creme or oil is always used as part of the massage, your body's complexion is treated to its own therapy: not only does the kneading increase circulation by bringing the blood supply close to the epidermis, but the heat it generates helps the creme penetrate the many layers of skin, leaving you feeling softer, silkier, free of dry, flaky patches. Massage is an all-around wonderful experience.

Meditation techniques such as TM (transcendental meditation) and Silva Mind Control, only two of the multitude of easily taught therapies for making yourself relax, can be the answer if you deal with stress all day long. They are more complicated than a jaunt to the gym—but sometimes one of these techniques is what's needed. Your bookstore has books on these therapies; many of which can be self-taught.

No matter how you achieve it, relaxation is without a doubt one of the best beautifiers around. When you learn to relax, you can stop tension headaches, lower-back pain caused by aggravation and even insomnia. You will experience a feeling of well-being, of being back in control. A real beauty has an aura of serenity and quietude about her. You too can have it. Inside and out.

CHAPTER 5

The Tan Commandments: The Best Care Under the Sun

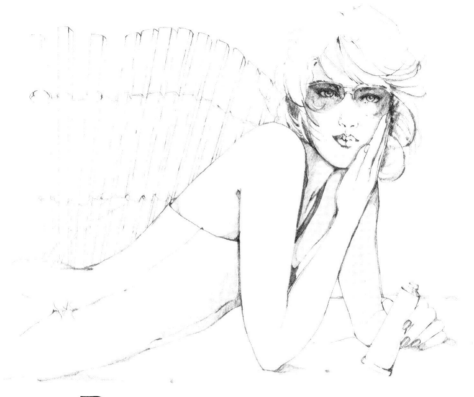

Do you know the story of how the tanning rage began?

After World War I there was an epidemic of tuberculosis in this country. Doctors would send their well-to-do patients in the north to warmer southern climates—Florida, California—to take in the sun and ward off the disease. Well, all too soon, being healthy became synonymous with having a suntan—it was just another status symbol for the wealthy. A tan meant you could afford to escape the northern cities and head south. The tan craze enabled Carl Fisher to found Miami Beach and start the pilgrimage to Palm Beach—the latter is still one of the most famous playgrounds of the rich.

The airlines capitalized on the Florida boom. My husband, Hal, used to write some of their advertising copy: "Have a millionaire's vacation on a piggybank budget!" Everyone, it seemed, was lured to Florida, and suckered, in my opinion, into getting a tan.

Unfortunately, unlike other popular American crazes, from the Hula Hoop to the maxi-coat, this one stuck with us, and with far-reaching consequences. It has taken four decades to make us realize that, far from being a sign of health, a suntan, and the more frequent and more harmful sunburn, is the body's warning system put into effect. And the message it tells your reflection in the mirror should be clear: Get out of the sun!

Weather Report

A good reporter is supposed to know the five Ws: Who, What, When, Where and Why. To get the real slant on the sun story, I'm going to answer all those questions for you.

THE WHAT AND THE WHY

What actually happens to your skin when it is burned or tanned is fascinating. Some doctors have made it their life's goal to explore these phenomena, but a basic understanding is certainly enough for us.

A sunburn and a suntan are two unrelated processes. A burn doesn't turn into a tan, though the light burn you suffered on day one might be slight enough to disappear in a couple of days, and the coloring process that the exposure also started off might have darkened into a tan by then.

A suntan is the body's defense against exposure to the sun, an attempt to limit the amount of damage to the skin by the powerful ultraviolet rays. After exposure, melanin, the pigment that accounts for the everyday tone of the skin, darkens, beginning the tanning process. Over the next few days, the body produces more melanin. This will darken the skin further. But if during this period your time in the sun exceeds the body's ability to produce melanin—if you stay out in the sun for a longer period than your skin can tolerate—you will burn, not tan.

Sunburn causes a more dangerous, more permanent reaction than tanning. The skin turns red as blood vessels dilate, causing the skin to smart. Unfortunately this discomfort isn't instantaneous, or you'd get out of the sun much sooner. Up to six hours can pass before the burn becomes very painful. Other symptoms like chills, headaches, blisters, can take up to twenty-four hours to peak. What happens is this: the epidermis thickens, causing that swollen, puffy look. If body fluids leak into the skin layers, blisters will form. These painful and unsightly burns can set the groundwork for a predisposition to skin cancers, which may develop after years of repeated exposure.

The burning process can start very quickly, after as few as five to ten minutes, depending on the melanin reserve inherent in your complexion. Those with very light, fair skin (read: little melanin) will burn right away. At the other extreme, those with brown or black skin tones can stay out the longest before burning, but will nonetheless burn eventually. And everyone suffers moisture loss right from the start.

Another shared effect of sun exposure is the long-range damage. The tan/burn appears to us to affect only the epidermis or the skin's surface; this is the acute, or short-lived, result of exposure. What the mirror doesn't show right away are the chronic or long-term effects, wrinkles forming from the very beginning in the dermis. Though they may not "surface" from the skin's activity center for five or ten years, those wrinkles, when they arrive, will be here to stay (unlike surface lines that result immediately and can be smoothed with your lubricant).

The long-range results are cumulative as well. One year's damage by ultraviolet rays that have penetrated the dermis builds on the next year's, and the next and the next. . . . Excessive and repeated exposure will inevitably cause premature signs of aging. After each burn, the skin expands, then as the burn subsides, it contracts, losing more elasticity each time, just like the rubber band that's been stretched over and over again.

This "solar elastosis," or sun-caused irreversible loss of elasticity, results whether you tan or burn (skin-preserving moisture is lost either way) and accounts for many of those signs of age we've playfully dubbed "crow's feet," "laugh lines," "furrows" and "squint" lines. It's not all that funny when your deep summer tan turns into deeper lines in the fall. If you doubt what I'm saying, bear this in mind:

As early as the age of twenty-five or thirty, your skin can look ten years older than it should. And after forty, you can double that. Believe me when I say that sunning is the worst thing you can do to your complexion.

THE WHO, THE WHERE AND THE WHEN

Who? Everyone!

As a general rule, the lighter the colors of your skin, eyes and hair, the more susceptible you are. The women of Celtic, Irish and Welsh descent are the most vulnerable.

All redheads and blondes must be very cautious. Yet those with an olive complexion, often accompanied by black hair, must still take care. Those with black skin tones generally have fewer skin problems—dark complexions have great levels of melanin, are often more resistant and have better healing ability than lighter complexions—but these, too, still burn. It was often thought that people living around the Mediterranean, like those in the Caribbean, had greater resistence to the sun than their northern neighbors. Yet Dr. Kate Mulopulos, Greece's first female dermatologist, has told me that skin cancers have become a problem in her country because of the strength of the sun and the local mania for having the deepest tan. She's trying to bring the lessons of sunsense to her countrymen so that they don't end up looking like those delicious, but wrinkled, Greek olives!

Your age plays a part in the sunburn process, too. Babies and children, though seemingly able to recover more quickly than adults, will burn faster than their parents because the ratio of their skin surface to body volume is greater and even one hour's damage can last a whole lifetime. Infants dehydrate and lose more perspiration faster, too. So baby your baby—and your young children as well, especially when they are outdoors all the time, oblivious to the need for protection. Start their sunsense today—and yours, too, if you haven't already.

WHERE? WHEREVER YOU GO!

You don't have to be in your swimsuit to be stung. Of course, the closer you are to the equator, the stronger the rays that reach you: you'll burn faster in the Bahamas than on a beach on Long Island Sound. You're more susceptible in higher elevations, too (Mexico City, for instance), because the screening atmosphere is thinner. But no matter where you are or what you're doing—driving, lunching at a sidewalk café, even walking the dog—you can get a burn, or at the least, suffer some skin-drying exposure. (Even the cement sidewalk you stroll on will reflect the sun's rays and bounce them all over you.)

Exercise caution at all times—and more of it than you think necessary. Did you know that the sand at the beach will reflect the sun, too? Even if you're sitting under an umbrella, 50 percent of its rays will reach you. And 100 percent of the rays will penetrate the water: always count swimming time as part of your total exposure and never swim unprotected by a sunscreen or sunblock (the sun and salt water have a lethal effect).

WHEN? ANYTIME!

You can expect the most devastating sun rays between 10:00 A.M. and 3:00 P.M. (11:00 to 2:00 is deadly!), yet a five o'clock afternoon sun can give you a burn, too.

Don't let the less-than-sunny days fool you. You can burn and blister on days that are gray, overcast, foggy, cloudy or hazy—the mist can even amplify damaging rays. Eighty percent of the UVs (ultraviolet rays) will reach your skin right through the clouds.

Don't let cool breezes and low temperatures get you off your guard. They give you a false sense of comfort and security and *zap!* the sunburn strikes.

THE ANSWER? PROTECTION!

You'll have to decide which is more important: a darker skin *tone* for summer or a softer, younger-looking *skin* year-round. Evaluate the risks and benefits of a tan. (If you already know what's best, see how you can fake a tan on page 88.)

When heading outdoors, arm yourself with sun products that protect. I wouldn't dream of staying inside to avoid the sun—the fresh air and outdoor exercise benefit my whole being too much for that. But I do it the right way—by preparing my skin first.

Product Report

There are three types of sun products available for your often different needs. Use them alone or in combination, as best suits your complexion characteristics. Remember that your face, even just the nose, may react differently from the rest of you.

Sunblock: to completely block all ultraviolet rays by deflecting them.

The product you choose must:

- completely stop tanning, burning, freckles, brown patches
- be completely water repellent so that you can go in and out of the water without worry, without reapplying
- be a tan regulator, allowing you to stop at any stage the tan you have acquired
- be opaque to deflect the burning rays yet blend with your complexion and minimize uneven skin tones (white masks are *out!*). Try my Sun Sensitive Creme.
- provide protection equal to 1-inch thickness of clothing
- contain zinc oxide to stop the burn of the shorter UV rays *and* PABA (para-aminobenzoic acid), a sunscreen that stops the tanning or longer UV rays.

Who needs a complete block? Those who are extremely sensitive to the sun; who burn right away; who are going to be outdoors for a great length of time; who are exposing skin for the first time (wearing a more revealing suit than usual, visiting a nudist beach or sunning on a private deck . . .); who will be outside longer than the recommended tanning time; who are prone to dry skin that lines easily.

Sunscreen: to permit varying degrees of UV rays to penetrate.

The product you choose must:
- contain chemicals that absorb the harmful rays
- include, along with a B vitamin, the most effective sunscreen
- remain effective in water (my Safer Tanning Formula, the most effective available, offers 90 percent protection for thirty minutes in water.

Who needs it? Those who have limited tolerance for the sun; who plan on extensive periods outdoors, especially when engaged in water sports; who are sensitive to the sun and burn after a short time, yet want to get a safe tan.

Suntan lotion: to tan without burning or peeling.

The product you choose must:
- contain some sunscreen agent (homo-menthyl salicylate is one of the best) to shield you from burning rays (like my Moisture Tan Creme)
- include very effective emollients to moisturize skin as it is tanning (lubricants comparable to those in your night creme/moisturizer)
- be frequently reapplied as this type of product will have limited screening effects

Who needs it? Those who want a tan and who tan easily (those with dark eyes especially)—you still need protection and lubrication; those who are outdoors a lot during the day (for reasons other than sunning) and who need protection against reflected rays (wear this as a moisturizer, alone or under makeup).

PRODUCTS *NEVER* TO USE

- cocoa butter
- baby oil (with or without iodine)
- coconut oil

You might as well grease a frying pan and jump in! They offer no protection, only a minimum of moisturizing ingredients.

THE TRUTH ABOUT THOSE SPF NUMBERS

- *Sun Protection Factor* numbers (2-15) are usually put there by the manufacturer, not a government agency

- They ask you to estimate the number of minutes it'll take you to burn (is that a test you'd willingly give yourself?)

- The numbers don't tell you if the product works in water, if it stops all pigment changes; only how long you can stay in the sun before burning if you use it

HOW TO GIVE YOURSELF A TAN CORRECTLY

1. Never go out in your bare summer clothes without protection. If you want to tan, apply your tanning lotion before going out —up to 20 minutes earlier to be sure it forms a seal.

2. If your skin is very sensitive, put on your first application of lotion after showering/bathing the night before, again in the morning.

3. Limit your first exposure to fifteen minutes. Add one third more time each day. If you're staying out after that time, apply a sunblock or sunscreen, depending on your sensitivity, or cover yourself (a terrycloth robe is good and fashionable; and a tightly woven straw hat and a block on your face to shield against reflected rays).

4. If using a sunscreen after exposure, reapply as needed. Unlike a sunblock, it won't last all day. Reapply after a half hour in the water; after a vigorous toweling; after excessive perspiration. Switch to a block if you are coloring too quickly.

5. Never try to get a tan in a day: you'll burn, peel and go home red instead of brown.

IRMA'S TAN COMMANDMENTS

For all vacation spots: sand, sun, sea and the slopes!

I. Thou shalt avoid sun exposure between 11:00 A.M. and 2:00 P.M.

II. Thou shalt carefully time sun exposure: fifteen minutes a day as a starter.

III. Thou shalt not be fooled by a cloudy day (the sun's rays can penetrate a light overcast or a haze and cause a bad burn).

IV. Thou shalt not feel protected by a beach umbrella (reflected sunlight from water or sand is frequently as strong as direct rays).

V. Thou shalt not feel immune to sunburn while snorkeling (rays also penetrate water).

VI. Thou shalt not mix medication and sun exposure. (The Pill can cause photosensitivity—brown spots and sunburn-like reactions. So can diuretics, tranquilizers, sulphonamides, and more. Consult your doctor if you're on medication.)

VII. Thou shalt never be fooled by a cooling breeze. (You may feel cool but a breeze sometimes may increase the burning effect of the sun's rays—the ultraviolet rays that cause all the trouble.)

VIII. Thou shalt rely only on suntan lotions that moisturize and remain on the skin *in* and *out* of water . . . otherwise you must reapply after swimming.

IX. Thou shalt remember that see-through clothing is no protection (if the sun's rays can penetrate, you might as well wear nothing).

X. Thou shalt never be beguiled by a deep tan today at the sacrifice of a good skin forever and a day.

HOW TO FAKE A SUNTAN WITH MAKEUP

· Use an instant-acting bronzing gel; work quickly, as it dries almost instantly. Remove before bed just as you would any makeup.

· Use a foundation in a dark shade; sponge it on for a natural look, taking care to bring it all the way to your clothing neckline.

· Use a blusher or bronzer on hands, legs, wherever you want to—for that healthy look of color, all over.

Sports Care: Protection Advice for Outdoor Activities

Biking. Hands and arms are especially prone to exposure. Wear long-sleeved clothing or apply a good sunscreen. Carry it with you for reapplication if needed. If weather is very sunny and hot, use a sunblock.

Gardening. Protect yourself as gardeners in Japan do, with gloves and tightly woven straw sun hats or umbrellas. Japanese women would never think of exposing their faces to the sun; they use a heavy, opaque white rice powder as protection; but here at home, a discreet sunblock is enough.

Golf. Wear gloves whenever possible. Use a visor to shield eyes, guard against expression lines. A sunblock on the lips and the back of the neck is advisable. Long, lightweight pants and shirt are also advisable; dark colors absorb more light.

Running. If weather permits, wear a lightweight sweatsuit to cover body and absorb perspiration. Use a sunblock on face, neck and hands. When bare-ing down, use sunscreen on exposed arms, legs and chest. In extreme heat, use a heavy lubricant around eyes, on lips (night creme is good).

Sailing/Boating. If you are careful about remembering to reapply, use a sunscreen. If not, use a sunblock right away—always if very sensitive and fair-skinned. The sun compares with salt water to easily damage skin, especially if skin is constantly wet; your products must contain heavy emollients, such as a mineral-oil complex or apricot-kernel oil.

Skiing/Snowmobiling. Protect against those doubly dangerous slopes: the snow reflects every bit of sun right at you; and you are more vulnerable to its rays because of the thinner atmosphere at those heights. Dress in several light layers so that you can peel one or two off as you get hot and still remain covered. Use a complex sunblock on all exposed areas, especially the lips. In very cold weather, wear a knit face mask, and a light application of moisturizer/night creme underneath.

Swimming. Use a sunblock if you'll be in the water for more than a half hour. Never scrimp on this protection: some of the worst sunburn cases were reported by school swim teams that neglected these precautions. The minimum: a water-repellant sunscreen; reapply frequently. Don't forget to protect your lips; and rinse off chlorine right away after leaving the pool.

Tennis. Sunblock is a must, as excessive perspiration will cause a sunscreen to wear off quickly. Wear a sweatband to keep sweat out of

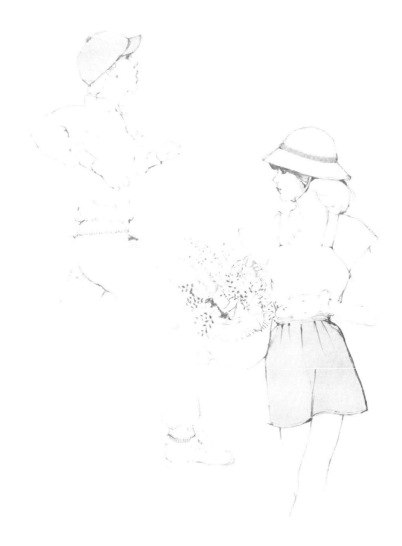

eyes, off face. Protect lips/eye area with moisturizer. Wear cotton shorts/top to absorb sweat, to keep sun product on longer. Avoid peak sunlight hours.

Walking. Wear sunglasses or a wide-brimmed hat to shield eyes. Replace your regular moisturizer with a suntan lotion if out all day. Apply it to exposed areas as you would body lotion.

A Lexicon of Sun Woes and Solutions

Blisters. *Sun blisters* appear when body fluids get trapped inside pores due to excessive heat, usually after a long first exposure. They can be very tiny and clustered in a group where there is skin friction (example: under the breasts) or they can be large and appear one by one. In most cases, they will subside in a few days and don't require any treatment—they're more annoying than dangerous. But blisters that occur as a result of a bad sunburn can be painful and can collect a great deal of fluid: these might need treatment by your doctor. To soothe blisters, treat as you would a sunburn (see below).

Fever blisters or *sores* can be more complex and are caused by a virus known as herpes simplex. Predisposition to this virus and an unprotected skin that's exposed to the sun accounts for these. The answer here is to use a total sunblock to prevent the sun from acting on your skin. If you aren't aware of having herpes simplex, yet think you might have gotten fever blisters, see your doctor for his diagnosis—this isn't something you can test yourself for.

Brown Patches. Technically known as chloasma, these blotches occur when persons who are taking certain drugs (the Pill, tetracycline, and a variety of others) are exposed to the sun's rays. These drugs give your skin a predisposition to photosensitivity, which results in the darkened areas. If you are on medication, ask your doctor if you might be photosensitive; if so, use a complete sunblock on all exposed areas while outdoors. One client of mine discovered brown spots on her hands and, after reviewing her daily schedule, realized that the window of her car reflected the sun onto her hands while she was driving. From then on, she wore either driving gloves or a sunblock. Use your body-brasing lotion and applicator gently over the blotched areas if these have already developed—this will help remove the blotches sooner.

NOTE: Brown spots, also known as liver spots, which appear, most often on hands, with advancing age, are not exclusively sun-related. Bleaches don't usually work. Old ideas are best: no bright nail polish or excessive jewelry that draws attention to hands, if you're bothered by the spots.

Freckles. Freckles that normally are too pale to notice will suddenly become apparent as melanin, the skin's pigment, darkens on first exposure to the sun. This often happens on the nose, the shoulders. . . . If you'd rather not have them, use a complete sunblock on susceptible areas—you know where they are. Once visible, they will disappear in a few days if you stop sunning or start using the block.

Heat Exhaustion. This occurs after long exposure to excessive heat, especially after a radical elevation in local temperature (when a cool sixty-degree day suddenly jumps to the eighties), or from too much strenuous activity in the sun accompanied by much perspiration. The symptoms (pale skin, rapid pulse, dizziness, nausea and even fainting) are caused by a loss of the body's salt through excessive sweating.

If this happens, slowly drink a glass of water in which a teaspoon of salt has been diluted and repeat once or twice more if necessary. Of course, get out of the sun, but stay warm. If you feel faint, sit down and put your head between your legs. Rest for at least thirty minutes; people have been known to think they've made a quick recovery, only to faint again upon standing.

Keratoses. These are raised, irregular brown growths that can occur on any exposed area of the body. They aren't skin cancers, but can precipitate them if not treated. Have any new or changed growths checked by your doctor, and removed if he or she suggests it. Also prevalent are *actinic keratoses*, small, scaly whitish patches. Do not dermabrase any suspect areas.

The best solution is prevention: limited exposure, maximum sun protection.

Peeling. This is one of the many disadvantages of tanning and burning. The sun speeds up the skin cycle, causing many layers of skin to die at once. Rather than flaking off imperceptibly, what looks like a thick layer peels off. Unless you moisturized as you tanned, there's no way to avoid this (and it's inevitable with a burn). After the fact, cremes won't stop it.

You can speed up the peeling by using your bodybrasing lotion twice a day—but be extra gentle, as the new skin underneath is very sensitive (it's being exposed before its time). Never start sunning again until the new skin is completely healed.

Skin Cancers. Known as carcinomas, these are frequently caused by overexposure to the sun, must be treated immediately (although the one redeeming feature of a skin cancer is that it rarely spreads beyond its margins when sun-related). They appear most often on those with very light skin. They are usually rough, irregular growths with a raised border and a central crater that can blister or bleed and scab.

Always have a skin cancer removed by a doctor after a proper diagnosis. If you have had one or more of these growths, you have a tendency toward them and should never go out in the sun without a complete, water-repellent sunblock. Forget about having a tan—it's just not worth the injury to your appearance and health.

Skin Irritations. A skin condition formally known as berloque dermatitis is another irritating result of sun exposure. Irregular discoloration in the form of dark brown spots occurs when sensitive skin that's been sprayed with fragrance, or with a sun product that contains fragrance, is exposed to the sun. The sun interacts with the chemicals or oils in the perfume/product and this interaction irritates the skin. I found this out one very hot and sunny day in Texas. I was wearing an off-the-shoulder blouse and had refreshed myself by splashing on cologne before going back into the heat. Well, the next morning, I woke with a large beige-colored blotch across one shoulder! Moral: Put fragrance on your clothing—not directly on skin that will be exposed to the sun (take care first that the fabric won't bleed). Finally, if you have sensitive or allergic skin, patch-test your sun products (especially those with PABA) on a small area of your body (keep the rest covered) to see if the sunscreen or block agent is irritating. If so, try other agents.

Sunburn. Ouch! But if you went out unprotected, or allowed your lotion to wear off, a sunburn is the unavoidable result. Try these remedies as needed:

1. Apply a soothing body balm (mine contains aloe because of its great healing properties). If the burn is slight, this should take the sting out. Avoid any of those spray-on preparations; the relief rarely lasts and the main ingredients can cause an allergic reaction.

2. Apply tepid compresses to the burned areas, dipping a soft cloth in the water and blotting it on skin, over and over.

3. If the burn is widespread, take a tepid bath. Mix in a handful of oatmeal—it is also soothing. Avoid any fragranced products, any soap. Pure talc afterward may help.

4. If the burn is severe, take two aspirin for its anti-inflammation properties. Aspirin will also relieve the headache that usually accompanies a lot of sun exposure.

5. If your eyes are red (you could have avoided this by wearing sunglasses that cut 65 percent of the sun's rays—you shouldn't be able to see your eyes through them in a mirror), keep the room dimly lit; don't try to read or watch TV.

6. If your lips are burned, treat them to a tepid compress, too. Then apply your night creme to prevent cracking.

7. Chills often follow a bad burn. Stay under a soft comforter or, if using blankets, keep a top sheet between them and you. Rest the entire evening—that's the only way the following days won't be lost to you!

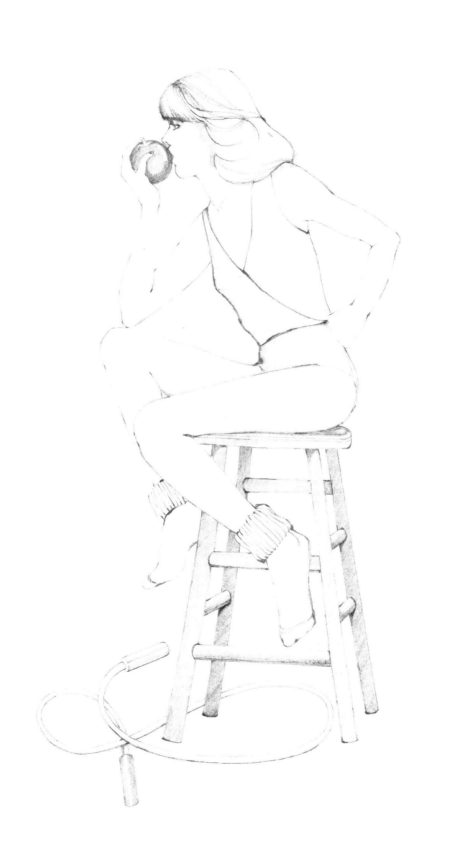

CHAPTER 6

Nourish and Invigorate: Your Diet and Exercise Program

G OOD nutrition and the proper exercise work wonders on your complexion, but the chain reaction includes a middleman: physical fitness—and that's what this chapter's about.

NUTRITION + EXERCISE = FITNESS → GREAT SKIN AND MORE!

Improving Overall Health

Fitness is a boon to your circulatory and respiratory systems. A fit heart means a stronger, more effective organ to pump blood at a slower (read: healthier) rate. The amount of blood that's pumped and the ability of the veins to carry it increase as well, resulting in greater circulation, which fuels the body (and complexion) with more of the oxygen the system was designed to carry. Your lungs function more efficiently, increasing the amount of air you can inhale with each breath. The complete chain benefits. (It also lags without fitness!)

An enhanced body system is better able to handle the demands you put on it, including the very exercise that strengthens it. The energy you draw on for exercise begets more energy; you won't be exhausted after a strenuous workout if you're fit. In fact, you feel more energized than before. And *less* hungry—you're too busy to think about eating (a boon to weight control or loss). Contrary to popular belief, you won't want or need as much food if you're fit, because the body uses its intake more efficiently—no more need to overfuel overtaxed organs. However, you will be able to eat more if you want to without gaining weight; you use more calories to maintain muscle, so the more muscle you have, the more you can eat.

Improving Your Figure

Achieving that universal goal, a slim figure, goes hand in hand with becoming fit. Here's how it is done.

Exercise. As the heart and all other muscles are developing, fat is being burned off within, and around them; the more you work your muscles, the more they use (and use *up!*) stored fat.

Diet. The quality as well as the quantity of food you eat is important—exercise alone won't make up for eating improperly. Raw, unprocessed foods are nourishing to the body. Processed, refined foods use up the body's resources just by being digested—they impart little or no value to the system. For optimum health, you need the healthiest diet; for weight loss as well, you'll have to limit your intake.

The combined balance of exercise and food—expenditure and intake—readjusts the body, reducing the percentage of fat, increasing the percentage of muscle. And that further increases fitness, too.

A Daily Diet

Until four years ago, I was eating the usual American diet: lots of meat, lots of refined carbohydrates (sugar- and flour-based foods). We all think that we are most fortunate because our standard of living (and eating) is high—we don't realize how confused we are. Yes, we have potentially the greatest abundance of food—but what we do with it is killing us. I had gotten deeper and deeper into the convenience-food game, not paying attention to nutrients, content to undo all neglect with a daily multivitamin—as if that could really make up for all the natural vitamins I was passing up by ignoring fresh foods.

And then, one summer, while spending a week at a friend's country house, everything changed for me, none of it planned (I didn't suddenly get a revelation the way people do during a therapy session—it was much more subtle). The weather was so hot that no one could bear the thought of eating a heavy meal, much less cooking one. We opted for salads—magnificent salads of the freshest vegetables and fruits. There

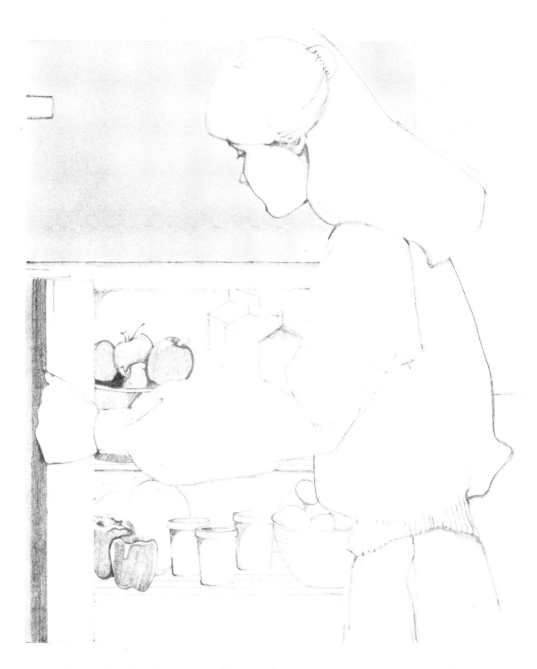

was such a selection that we could vary the menu—from a green salad with a dozen artfully sliced vegetables tossed in, to a simple combination of berries, sweet and succulent. Without my being led into this as a "sensible" change of diet, it happened as a natural course of events. I found that I simply felt better (no one had to put the suggestion into my head) without meats, heavy oils and sauces.

OUR ESSENTIAL NUTRIENTS	USED BY THE BODY FOR	FOUND IN THESE RECOMMENDED FOODS
protein	cell renewal and repair, the body's basic building blocks	chicken, turkey, fish, eggs, dairy products
carbohydrates	energy and heat	foods that come from the ground: vegetables, fruits, wheat and grains
fats	support and protection of organs, nerves, absorption of vitamins A, D, E	nuts and seeds, dairy products, vegetable/seed/nut oils
vitamin A	vision; healthy tissues	apricots, carrots, green leafy vegetables, dairy products
vitamin B: B 1 (thiamine)	nervous system; digestion	whole grains, rice, nuts and seeds
B 2 (riboflavin)	iron absorption; digestion	dairy products, wheat germ
B 3 (niacin)	general health	poultry, fish, whole grains, nuts and seeds
B 5 (pantothenic acid)	nervous system; digestion; proper growth	egg yolks, nuts, legumes (peas and beans)
B 6 (pyridoxine)	" "	whole grains, wheat germ, rice, bananas
B 12 (cyanocobalamin)	development of red blood cells; good metabolism	seafood, eggs
biotin	absorption of other nutrients	egg yolks, dairy products, nuts, whole grains
choline	liver function; conversion of fat to energy	egg yolks, whole grains, green vegetables

(continued on page 99)

OUR ESSENTIAL NUTRIENTS	USED BY THE BODY FOR	FOUND IN THESE RECOMMENDED FOODS
folic acid	red blood cells; nervous system	legumes, leafy green vegetables, whole grains
inositol	circulation; used with choline for healthy arteries	legumes, wheat germ
PABA (para-aminobenzoic acid)	healthy skin; protection against sunburn	brown rice
vitamin C	protection against infection; strong bones and teeth	citrus fruits, tomatoes, green and red bell peppers, strawberries, papaya, green leafy vegetables
vitamin D	healthy bones and teeth; absorption of calcium	sunshine, fortified milk, tuna, salmon
vitamin E	preserving the other vitamins	vegetable oils, whole wheat and other grains, asparagus, spinach
the basic minerals:		
copper	formation of hemoglobin	whole grains, green leafy vegetables
calcium	healthy teeth and bones	dairy products
iodine	healthy thyroid	shellfish
iron	strong blood cells	wheat germ, fish, legumes, egg yolks
magnesium	synthesis of protein, fat and carbohydrates	whole grains, nuts, soybeans, vegetables
potassium	cardiovascular system	bananas, potatoes, nuts, grains
sulphur	healthy hair, skin, nails	protein foods, whole wheat, legumes
zinc	general health, fast healing	shellfish, wheat germ

Looking back, I think I was always a closet vegetarian. That week in the country only confirmed my suspicions. The thought of steak never made my mouth water—and when I learned that charcoal-broiling was a dangerous cooking method, I gave it up. In fact, the very idea of raw meat makes me uncomfortable, too, due, no doubt, in part to my first cooking experiences as a newlywed. When Hal and I were just starting out, we had to watch every cent. I was at the supermarket one day and was very impressed with the sale on chickens—a very low price for an "undressed" bird. Being new to kitchen duties, I had little idea of what the qualification meant, and as the wrapper was opaque, it wasn't until I returned home with my fabulous bargain that I discovered my dinner's main course was wearing its head, feet and tail—feathers and all! Well, I ran out of the kitchen as fast as I could and waited for Hal to come home and pluck it!

Fortunately I learned to buy my poultry dressed, and, more fortunately, I learned to eat it in moderation. It's the only "flesh" I eat, except for fish, and usually only when I'm eating out. My favorite protein sources are nuts and dairy products. It's not really high levels of protein we need but *carbohydrates* in their natural state: vegetables, fruits and whole grains like buckwheat (kasha), bran and barley. Without the energy supplied by carbohydrates, the body would use its own protein, and that's bad since protein's chief function is repair. Fats are needed, too, especially for the digestion and absorption of the fat-soluble vitamins, A, D and E; they are stored in the body along with its fat reserves and don't need daily resupplying. Fats are inherent in nuts and dairy products, so I often leave out butter, cream and the like—all the refined fats.

In addition to carefully regulating what I eat, I watch amounts. I've found that 800 calories a day are plenty for me (here I stress that this is what I recommend for myself alone) because I am very thin and small-boned. It's the amount I stick to to avoid gaining—you too can do that once you know your daily requirement. (I'll tell you how to find that out soon.) Our daily calorie requirements, like the indications on most weight charts, are too high, especially for women over twenty-five. Yes, I agree that teenagers and pregnant women need more, but most other women need less, closer to ten calories per pound each day than the often recommended fifteen. No matter how high-pressured or high-level your job, whether you're an active mother and homemaker or an executive or both, the energy most often expended is mental, not physical. The physical energy expended in running to make a bus or driving the kids to school is not great in terms of caloric demands. Mental rest—more sleep at night or a midday nap—is the answer, not more calories.

Here's how I break up my daily calorie intake:

Breakfast: usually small, definitely some citrus. Grapefruit in the morning does something great for my metabolism all day. I'm a firm believer in it. For protein, I'll have a small amount of nuts or grains or a soft boiled egg.

Lunch: I hardly ever eat more than a green salad—its the greatest because you can keep eating and eating it (as long as you don't heap on the dressing). Chef's salads and Niçoise salads also supply essential protein because they include tuna, cheese or lean meats. I like lunch to be quick, not a time-consuming waste. I don't believe in lingering over the meal with a few glasses of wine—though if you require many more calories than I do, now is the time to have them because calories you consume at lunch are burned off more readily than those in your food and drink at night.

Dinner: I enjoy eating at night and that's a pleasure I've had to curb. Night calories turn into fat, so I keep my eating simple: raw or steamed vegetables, a handful of nuts or maybe cottage cheese, broiled poultry or fish or an assortment of fruits. If you're a night eater, make the switch to an earlier time gradually. First, cut back during the day to avoid gaining more weight during the transition. Next, start by reducing your after-six eating by 100 calories each week. Add those calories to lunch or breakfast. Continue this 100-calorie-a-week transposition until your night calories are only one third to one quarter of your daily intake.

You can see how carefully I have planned my day after taking into account my eating patterns and my calorie limit. This is something you can do for yourself. Answer these questions on a piece of paper.

· Do you like a full breakfast that will keep you satisfied until lunch or later? Do you prefer not eating until mid-morning?
· Are you really hungry at night or do you eat dinner out of habit or because you think your family needs this heavy meal? (With a hot school lunch, your kids will be better off with an afternoon snack of fruit and nuts and a lighter dinner.)
· Do you get hungry during the day and snack? (Mini-meals spread out over the day will keep you satisfied around the clock, and away from empty-calorie sweets.)

· Do you get very hungry at night? (Filling up on high-volume, low-calorie salads will answer your needs without weight gain if you find it impossible to change your eating habits.)

· When, during the day and/or night do you have the most time to eat carefully? (You should schedule hearty meals when you have time for them; fill in with portable goodies like nuts and raisins.)

Now look at your answers and map out an eating schedule accordingly; when to eat, which meals to concentrate on. Establish a pattern to suit your needs and get used to it; it's not just for losing weight, it's for every day.

Diet Dilemmas

PROBLEM: *Calorie Counting*

SOLUTION: I've found that using calories as a measure of how much you can eat is very helpful. Yes, it can be time-consuming, but only until you get the hang of it. After a few weeks of learning what 40 calories of carrots looks like, etc., it becomes second nature. And when you're always conscious of maintaining your weight, second nature is really how it has to be.

To find out how many calories you need, determine how many you usually eat in a day. Write everything down and look up each portion measured by ounces to find how many calories it contains. Total up. Do this for a week, weighing in every morning. Now ask yourself if you gained or maintained or lost. The rest is elementary: if you lost, you ate too little (great if you're trying to lose); if you stayed the same, perfect (now start using the calorie allotment more wisely); if you gained, cut back (a one-pound gain means 500 calories too many was eaten every day for seven days because one pound of weight is the cumulative result of 3,500 calories of unused intake).

NOTE: if you want to lose, cut back your maintenance level by 500 calories a day. This will net you a one-pound loss a week. Remember: Slow and steady wins the race.

PROBLEM: *Vitamins*

SOLUTION: It's hard to know when you've gotten all the vitamins you need out of the foods you eat. How long the carrot traveled to reach you has a lot to do with how many of its original nutrients were left when you got around to eating it. Even less satisfactory are the vitamins you get from a pill—one multivitamin pill barely covers the minimum requirement set by the government. Many nutritionists say this is far too low. The result is that we often make haphazard guesses, and that's not good either.

To make a better choice, ask yourself how you feel on your present diet. If you don't like your answer, improve your food selection. Buy produce the day you will eat it, not in advance (yes, that means daily stops at the store, but the few extra minutes it takes on your way home from another errand is worth it). Buy produce from a fruit and vegetable store or, if you live in the country, from a local farmer. Buy what's in season or what's flown in freshest. Never buy packaged produce you can't select yourself (supermarkets are notorious for choosing for you).

If you're still not satisfied, see your doctor. A blood test can determine any vitamin deficiencies and you can chart the proper course knowledgeably.

PROBLEM: *Bad Habits and Addictions*

SOLUTION: Learning to be satisfied with one piece of chocolate or a small portion of ice cream was the hardest for me. But it was a must: I had to indulge myself every now and then, but because I knew it was "bad" for me, I was determined not to go overboard. If you question every little thing you eat, you can really take the fun out of life: regulated cheating is okay—not great, but if it takes a little of that to stay on the right track most of the time, then it's worth it.

The worst bad habits are the addictive ones: coffee, tea, chocolate, sodas, alcohol. Try water, fruit juices (diluted to save calories), lemonade made with artificial sweetener, skim milk. Give up martinis for a cocktail of sparkling water and lime—eat the lime slice as I do.

PROBLEM: *Junk Foods*

SOLUTION: Understand why they aren't any good (they supply no nutritive value, no vitamins, only calories and the grease that does nothing for the complexion). Give them up for one month. When you bite into your next hot dog, after a month of eating fresh fruits, vegetables, salads and other unadulterated foods, you may just find that the hot dog is not as delicious as you once thought.

PROBLEM: *Losing Weight*

SOLUTION: I don't believe in seesawing up and down in weight as you alternately diet and go off your diet. This stretches the skin, causing it to lose elasticity. Nor do I believe in being on a perpetual diet, never

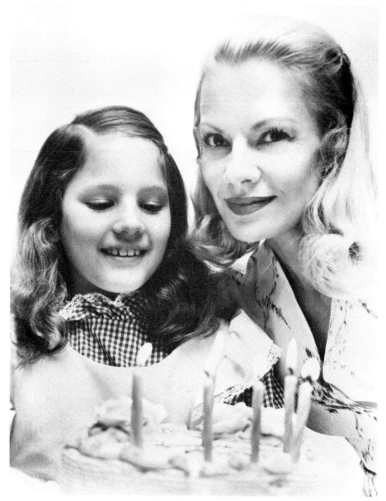

Good eating habits are a must—but an occasional slice of Stacey's birthday cake is an irresistible treat!

really losing weight, but boring everyone around you with incessant talk about it. What I do believe in is a permanent change in eating habits— something you can get accustomed to over a long period of time—that will insure you don't ever gain back more than two or three pounds, say, after a vacation. I know it's hard to believe when you're in the doldrums, but with time and a change in habits, you can accomplish more than you ever dreamed.

Until I changed the way I was eating, I was likely to gain five pounds or more after a binge, and I was driving myself crazy on a variety of diets. As I indicated before, I'm not the type of person who is satisfied with just one bite of ice cream—I have to have the whole container, and then I feel guilty for hours afterward. If I'm out for dinner and I indulge in a rich dessert, that too can start me off. I'll come home full, but craving more sweets, any I can find: candy, cookies, you name it. Before you know it, there's my five pounds. You may not think that's a lot, but on someone as small as I am, five pounds can look like fifteen!

To stop the cycle, even after I was on a diet that consisted mainly of salad, I had to moderate my sweet tooth. I said to myself one day that it had to be just as easy to have good habits as bad. And let's face it, we weren't born loving lemon meringue pie—it was an acquired taste, one I could un-acquire. I reasoned that I was crazy to undo all the good of my high-quality diet by binging on desserts and I made up my mind to learn to be satisfied with one slice of pie now and then, for both my figure and my health.

I know that this sounds a lot easier than it is—I readily admit it wasn't easy for me and still isn't. I know, too, that you can be so depressed about weight that you can hardly do anything about it. It's a natural reaction for a woman who has to cook dinner for four every night, go out twice a week for restaurant meetings and is already twenty pounds too heavy. But depression isn't the final answer—it's the stage you reach right before you pull yourself up and say, I've had it with my weight, I'm not going to spend the rest of my life as a fat person, I'm going to take it off. Once you make up your mind and get yourself motivated, you'll have only the most minor problems (plateaus, urges) along the way, and you can handle them all.

There are two ways to approach new habits and weight loss:

1. Start eating the right foods to improve your health without worrying about weight loss—eat nuts instead of cake, steamed brown rice and vegetables instead of a pork chop. Use the following diet as a guide, but increase the portions specified if you are still hungry. (Don't use this leeway as an excuse to gain, however!) After two to four weeks, when you feel comfortable with the new foods, gradually limit quantities until your portions equal those outlined below.

2. Start the diet immediately to bring down your weight as you get accustomed to the new foods. After an initial loss of up to ten pounds (depending on your figure needs), maintain your new weight by increasing the portions somewhat and adding sensible amounts of wholesome foods. Don't replace the food suggestions with equal-calorie but lower-nutrition substitutes like sweets and creams. After three weeks, go back on the weight-loss diet if you need to. (Learning to maintain a loss in stages helps keep off those pounds by letting your body adjust to their loss.)

IRMA'S SEVEN-DAY WEIGHT LOSS DIET

		calories
MONDAY		
breakfast:	1 grapefruit and 1 orange, sectioned	200
lunch:	8 ounces cottage cheese sprinkled with 1 tablespoon wheat germ, served in half a cantaloupe	320
dinner:	crudité plate: 1 sliced carrot, 6 asparagus tips, 6 mushroom caps, 6 cherry tomatoes, green pepper rings	70
	6 ounces brown rice, weighed cooked, steamed with herbs	200
snack:	15 almonds and 1 ounce sunflower seeds	200
		990
TUESDAY		
breakfast:	6 ounces grapefruit juice	65
	1 cup kasha with ½ cup skim milk	150
lunch:	fresh vegetable or minestrone soup	80
	spinach salad with mushrooms and 1 sliced egg, boiled (unlimited spinach, mushrooms)	100
	1 cup fresh pineapple, cut in small sections and tossed with berries	80
dinner:	4 ounces steamed striped bass	120
	1 stuffed potato: baked, scooped out and mixed with a little scallion, chopped fine and some chopped fresh dill or parsley, slid under broiler until top is browned	75
	2 cups steamed cauliflower or broccoli	60
snack:	1 large banana	100
		830
WEDNESDAY		
breakfast:	½ large papaya stuffed with a sliced kiwi fruit	150
	1 slice whole wheat bread with 1 teaspoon butter	100

(continued on page 107)

WEDNESDAY		calories
lunch:	2 ounces Swiss cheese melted on 4 thick slices of tomato, ½ ounce on each slice	240
	8 ounces zucchini and carrot sticks	40
dinner:	chicken broth	15
	salad plate: romaine lettuce (as much as you want) with chopped red cabbage, red onion slices and endive spears with dressing of 1 tablespoon red-wine vinegar with fresh herbs (chives, basil, dill)	
	3 ounces cubed chicken	280
	1 cup strawberries	50
snack:	a red bell pepper cut in rings or strips	15
		890

THURSDAY		
breakfast:	1 cup bran cereal, ½ cup skim milk, 1 banana	250
	4 ounces orange or grapefruit juice	40
lunch:	cottage cheese (4 ounces) surrounded by 20 grapes, 2 peaches (4 ounces each), ½ cup blueberries and 5 large cashew nuts	350
dinner:	steamed vegetables: 3 cups spinach topped with 1 medium zucchini, grated, ¼ cup green peas and ½ onion	100
	2 ounces roast beef	120
	1 medium baked potato with fresh chives and pepper	100
snack:	8 ounces tomato juice with seasonings	70
		1,030

FRIDAY		
breakfast:	oatmeal (1 ounce measured dry) with cinnamon, ½ cup skim milk	150
	8 ounces grapefruit juice	80
lunch:	Spanish omelet: 2 eggs filled with fresh tomato sauce (1 tomato, puréed, simmered with ½ chopped green pepper, ½ chopped onion and desired spices)	200

(continued on page 108)

FRIDAY   calories

dinner: 3 ounces stir-fried chicken that has marinated
           for 30 minutes in soy or teriyaki sauce,
           cooked in the sauce and a little chicken
           broth, with scallions, bean sprouts, pea pods,
           water chestnuts and ½ onion (vegetables
           totaling 16 ounces)   300
           1 pear or 2 small peaches   75
snack: 5 walnuts   100
                                                                    ─────
                                                                      905

SATURDAY

breakfast: in blender, whirl 4 ounces orange juice, ½
           cup berries, ½ cup pineapple and 3 ice cubes
           until ice is dissolved   130
lunch: sun salad: top 4 cups spinach with ½ ounce
           shredded cheese, 1 cup chopped grapefruit
           sections, ½ ounce each of sunflower seeds
           and raisins, and cashews or almonds   350
dinner: 8 ounces lobster meat with lemon   200
           4 ounces string beans   25
           1 cup cherries   100
snack: salad of watercress and 12 cherry tomatoes   75
                                                                    ─────
                                                                      880

SUNDAY

breakfast: ½ Spanish melon   60
           15 almonds   100
*lunch/
dinner:*   3 ounces whole wheat pasta, weighed
           before cooking, topped with fresh tomato
           sauce (see Friday lunch)   350
           mixed green salad with dressing (see
           Wednesday dinner)   130
evening: 1 large pear, sectioned, topped with ½ cup
           crushed raspberries   150
snack: 10 medium-sized boiled shrimps
           (about 4 ounces)   100
                                                                    ─────
                                                                      890

NOTES ON THE DIET

1. The daily calorie allotment is a median number for losing 1 pound a week; some women can lose more eating 900 calories a day, some less. Because I've given you individual calorie counts, you can adjust the diet to your needs: add or subtract 100 to 300 calories a day.

Example: if you're losing too slowly, cut your lunch portion in half or eliminate the snack.

2. Eat only what's listed. If a salad doesn't call for dressing, don't use any. You can have coffee or tea, though I recommend cutting back, but don't add sugar, milk, cream or non-dairy creamer—you get the idea.

3. If you want to vary the menus after the first week, make honest substitutions: honeydew for cantaloupe, yogurt for cottage cheese, hazelnuts for almonds, tuna for shrimp, Bibb lettuce for Boston—*not* a slice of pound cake for the pasta, *not* a steak for the sun salad.

4. Give yourself a chance. Wait two weeks before looking at the scale. You'll be losing weight slowly and your body fluids can rise up to three pounds a day, masking your loss, discouraging you if you get on the scale too soon. Let the fit of your clothes be your guide—a far more accurate test of weight loss. Above all, weigh yourself only on your own scale—scales can vary a lot, and what you don't need is to get on a friend's and see a five-pound gain!

HOW TO COPE WHILE LOSING WEIGHT

· Dieting on the road can be especially difficult. Certain trips are fun, even business trips, but as a steady "diet" I find them to be terrible for the spirit and for beauty. Half the time I am out promoting so much I don't know where I am!

I try to avoid tempting, overly rich restaurant meals by bringing my own meals along: I bring foods that can be munched out of hand such as: nuts, raisins, fruits, whole wheat crackers, even string beans.

· Dieting when you must eat at restaurants is tricky.

1. Find out the type of meals served before you decide on the place—stay away from "cream-based" restaurants.

2. Explain to the chef, perhaps earlier in the day by phone, the restrictions of your diet and ask what he recommends. A good restaurant will be more than willing to cater to you. After all, isn't that why you go out?

3. Don't drink any wine or liquor—these are really useless calories.

Feel you need a drink in your hand? Order club soda (if you don't like it, you don't have to drink it, but it's there for security). Don't slather bread with butter. Don't eat the bread unless it's freshly made and hearty: raisin pumpernickel, fresh rye or whole wheat bread—all are very popular today.

· Shopping for food is the most difficult chore. Learn which are the lower-calorie brands of the foods you like. Most often that means fresh rather than canned or frozen. Use the supermarket for household staples (paper goods, laundry products and mineral water). For produce, visit a greengrocer. For seafood, the fish store; for lean chicken or turkey, the butcher; for fresh nuts and grains, perhaps a local bakery or health-food store.

> If you're going to use condiments on a maintenance diet (ketchup, mayonnaise, etc.) see if you can make them yourself, eliminating the additives packaged products almost always have.

> Never buy the diet-pack cans of vegetables or fruits. They are over-priced, over-chemicaled, and don't even taste real. Buy only seasonal fresh fruits and vegetables; they're the least expensive, the most nutritious and the tastiest!

> Don't go to the supermarket hungry: the food will look better to you than it is (even the pictures on frozen foods will drive you nuts).

> When you must go to the supermarket, stay out of the aisles that tempt you: ice-cream section, baked goods, candies, etc.

> Don't make your kids the scapegoats for your cheating. I once tried telling myself I was buying ice cream for my daughter—well, the flavor was coffee, my favorite, while she prefers strawberry. Why encourage bad habits in our kids—maybe they aren't overweight, but are they healthy enough? And how are their dental bills?

· Pamper yourself to reduce the boredom of dieting. Lobster, shrimp, crab—that's my idea of a diet! Enjoy these low-calorie delicacies every now and then, add a vegetable and a salad and you have a meal fit for a queen.

· Cook as little as possible. Eat raw salads, and other fresh handy foods as much as possible. Fix a gigantic bowl of raw vegetables (leave out the lettuce as it quickly wilts) and eat at will with minimal preparation time. The less preoccupied with food you are, the easier it will be to limit your intake.

· Drink plenty of water to fill you up, flush your system of burned fats. Have a glass with each meal, and more in between. Remember your body works best when hydrated.

· If you get hungry between meals, divide your intake into 6 mini-meals. Have part of breakfast at 9, the rest at 11. Lunch at 1, a snack at 3, your dinner salad or vegetable at 5, the rest at 7. This shrinks the stomach and the desire for calorie-laden meals, and reduces the inclination to over-eat. It's a good system for anyone with a stomach ailment or digestion problem: a mini-meal won't tax the digestive tract, leaves you with fewer calories to burn at one time.

· Know your weaknesses. I love raisins, can rarely be trusted with them—and though they are great nutritionally, they are very high in calories. So I usually avoid them. I have a friend with a worse sweet tooth than mine. She loves desserts, but swears off them while losing weight. Even if she topples her calorie limit with a big entree at a restaurant, she won't break her no-dessert rule and resists starting the sweet chain reaction. The next day, she has no trouble resuming her dieting schedule.

IF YOU LOVE IT, KEEP IT OUT OF THE HOUSE

· To lose the weight you'd like to and, more importantly, the bulges, you have to combine your food consciousness with an effective exercise plan—there are no two ways about it. Yes, with diet alone, you will notice some loss, primarily on the scale. But if you want the results you'll be able to see in the mirror, nude or with clothes on, you have to work off those inches through physical exertion.

You'll also have to be patient, though the inches will come off in less time than it took to put them there. Realistically, expect three weeks of a daily program—ten minutes a day—to pass before the tape measure shows results. There are no gimmicks involved, no magic spell to cast—just some hard work.

To be physically fit, as well as svelte, add to these ten minutes another fifteen, every other day, of active sport that works the heart and lungs—*aerobic* exercise. There are many different sports to choose from, but they all work to strengthen the heart by increasing its rate, the number of strokes it beats per minute, during the exercise. This brings about a lower, healthier heart rate the rest of the time.

Note: It's important to know when to stop losing weight. Often the only way you'll know is if people tell you. Most of us are too subjective about how we look to evaluate this properly. I once got down to eighty-five pounds—to what I thought was my ideal weight —only to be hit with a slew of negative reactions. Everyone who saw me thought I was under the weather. (The ten pounds I was able to put back on were the most satisfying!)

Daily Exercise: Alternatives Eliminate Drudgery

For me, exercise has no redeeming feature—except the fantastic way it makes me look and feel. But, oh, having to do it every day—that's the disadvantage. As with everything else, we want results with very little effort. That's impossible. But exercise can be made more palatable, depending on the route you take.

Calisthenic-type exercises are a must for improving muscle tone. I like to get them out of the way first thing in the morning so that I don't have to worry about doing them at night. But any time of the day is good, as long as you do them each day. Follow the ones I do or get a cassette that will "talk" to you if you prefer. Some people need real prodding—in person. For them, the gym is a wise investment—once they pay for a membership, they go.

Aerobic-type exercises are a must for improving your most important organ, the heart. These can be done on your own or at the gym, if it offers the needed equipment. Working out three times a week, combining an aerobic and a calisthenic program, can eliminate the morning routine I follow. The combination is up to you.

Now for the specifics to get you going.

If you're out of condition, start slowly, using the at-home exercises first, and only after an okay from your doctor. Your next office visit will be a good time to discuss your changes in diet, too.

IRMA'S EIGHT EXERCISES TO GET
YOU READY FOR YOUR DAY

1. MINI-PUSH-UPS

Lie flat on your stomach, arms bent at the elbows, palms flat on the floor near each shoulder, legs bent at the knees, heels reaching to your buttocks.

Keeping your back straight, push up until your arms are straight. From your head through your torso to your knees, your body should form a straight raised line.

Slowly lower to the floor.

Repeat four more times, building up to a total of ten.

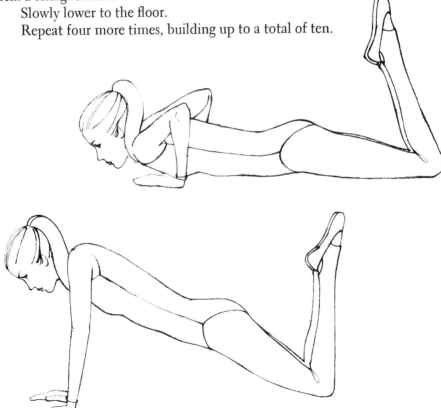

2. MINI-SIT-UPS

Lie on your back, your hands behind your head, knees bent, feet flat on the floor. Inhale.

Exhale and curl up, starting from the head: lift head, neck, shoulders and upper back.

Inhale as you relax to the floor.

Exhale and repeat four more times, working up to a total of ten.

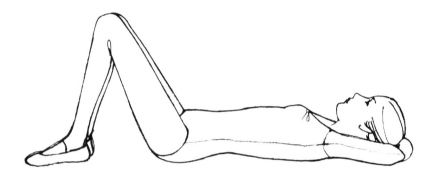

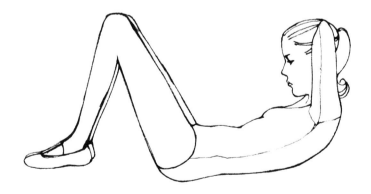

3. LEG-UPS

Lie flat, hands behind your head, legs extended. Inhale.

Exhale and slowly raise your legs until they form a right angle with your body.

Inhale and slowly lower your legs.

Exhale and repeat four more times working up to a total of ten.

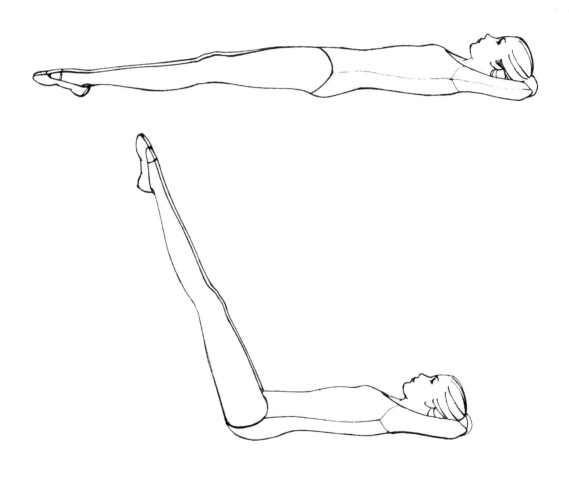

4. CRUNCHES

Lie flat as in the previous exercise. Inhale.

Exhale and slowly curl up from the head, bringing your knees to your chest as your back lifts off the floor.

Inhale as you relax to the floor.

Exhale and repeat four more times, working up to a total of ten.

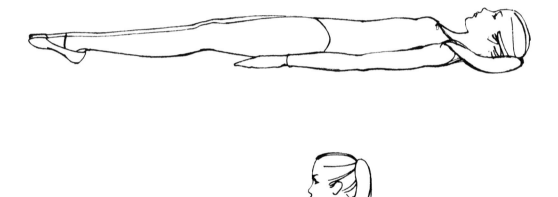

5. DONKEY KICKS (not a flattering name, but they work!)

Kneel on all fours, hands flat in front of you, shoulder-width apart, head up. Inhale.

Exhale and bring your right knee toward your forehead.

Inhale and extend the right leg behind you, until it is straight, parallel to the floor, but elevated (don't let the foot drop).

Exhale and bring your knee back toward your forehead.

Repeat the exercise four more times, working up to a total of ten for each leg.

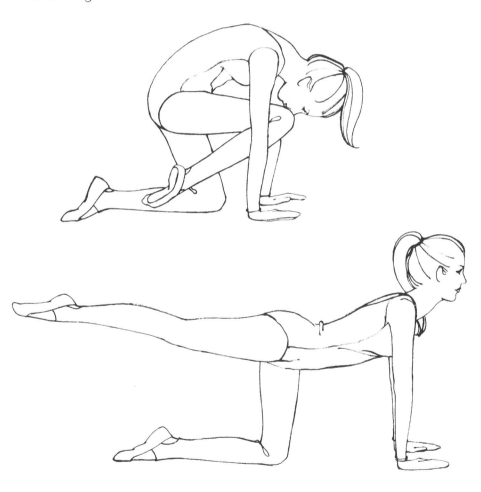

6. Single Leg Raises

Lie on your left side, body flat, head in your left palm, right hand at your waist for support, and bend your left leg in toward your chest. Inhale.

Exhale and raise your right leg to a 45-degree angle with the floor, no higher, always keeping it straight.

Breathing regularly, circle the straight leg forward, making five large circles.

Then make five large circles in the opposite direction.

Lower the leg and repeat the exercise on the other side.

Build up to ten circles in each direction, for each leg.

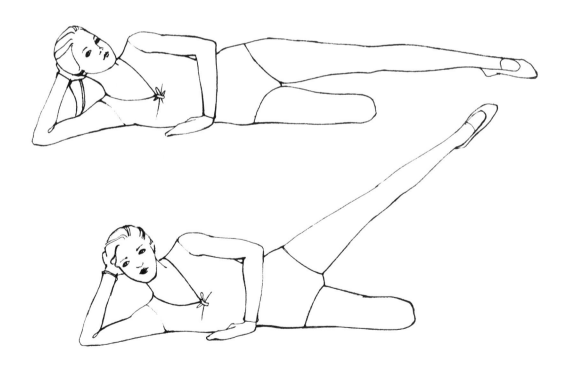

7. Double Leg Raises

Lie on your left side as in the previous exercise, but with both legs straight.

Raise the right leg to a 45-degree angle and hold it there, using a chair or a low table for support if needed. Inhale.

Exhale and lift the lower leg so that your heels touch—without lowering the top leg at all.

Inhale and lower the bottom leg only.

Repeat four more times, then repeat the exercise on the other side.

Build up to ten lifts on each side.

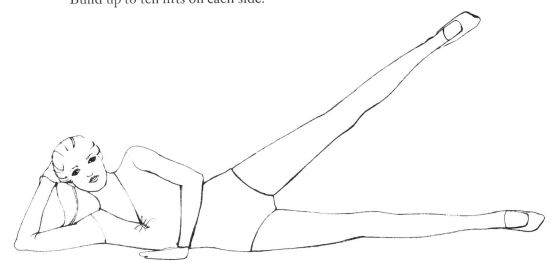

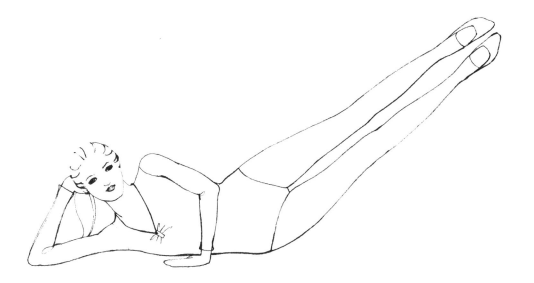

8. REAR LEG RAISES

Lie flat on your stomach, hands under your hipbones so that each palm cups the bone of each joint. Inhale.

Without lifting the hips off the floor, raise the right leg as high as you can as you exhale, slow and steady.

Inhale and lower the leg.

Repeat four more times, then repeat the exercise with the left leg.

Work up to ten lifts with each leg.

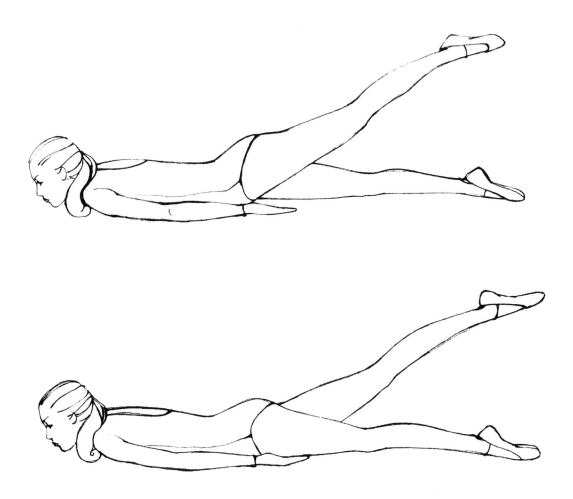

APPROVED ALTERNATIVES

To do at home:

· Ask your doctor to evaluate your needs and prescribe an individualized program of exercises for you.
· Have a professional gym instructor test your strengths and weaknesses and devise a workout routine.
· Buy a pre-recorded exercise cassette or tape and follow its instructions.
· Follow along with a televised exercise show, often carried by cable TV networks—often more than once a day—to adapt to your schedule.

To do away from home:

· Join a fully equipped gym to alternate your program as you like: combine aerobics with classes in calisthenics and/or yoga; swim; work out with progressive endurance machines (these are weight-lifting machines whose resistance can be increased as you strengthen muscles).
· Start a dance-exercise, yoga or ballet program at a school specializing in one of these; attend individual classes two or three times a week.
· Indulge in private-instruction classes, usually held in the teacher's home or studio; classes are small and may even be one to one.

How to Decide on a Gym/School/Class

Decide on what you are willing to pay. Joining a gym can represent a yearly investment of three hundred to five hundred dollars, but that should entitle you to attend every day, for as long as you like each time. Going to an exercise class can cost seven to ten dollars per session, and over a year's time, attending twice a week, you'll spend quite a bit more than the gym would cost, though paying by the week may be easier.

Ask yourself how much luxury you want: a ballet school might get you a class with a barre and little else; a full-facility gym will have private lockers, showers, a sauna—but the school can charge significantly less. Don't overlook the Y. Many branches have excellent facilities at reasonable prices.

Determine the convenience you need: does your exercise place have to be near work (if you go during lunch, for instance)? Or should it be nearer home (for evenings and the weekends)? A gym that involves both travel time and money will be a waste. Determine the hours most convenient for your workout and ask about their schedules right away: the two must coincide. Optimally a gym should be open long enough to satisfy any last minute schedule changes. Twice-weekly group or individual instruction classes will have one set time that you'll agree upon up front.

Investigate thoroughly before plunking down any money (the most reliable operations will have contracts that offer your money back if you're not satisfied within a certain period of time). Visit at a peak hour (lunchtime if in a business district, Sunday morning, if residential). Is everyone congenial? Are there enough staff members to go around? Are the surroundings pleasant and clean (that will begin to mean a lot soon) even if the facilities are plain? Don't be afraid to ask members for an honest evaluation—this will also tell you if fellow exercise devotees are friendly. (Of course, you're going there to work, but the atmosphere should be relaxed.)

Ask for a trial run. Some places will let you sit in on a class; others will only offer a tour of the premises. There's nothing wrong with this: if you like the place, offer to pay for one visit and then make your determination.

Even if you follow your morning at-home exercises faithfully, don't rule out professional, personalized instruction. After going to Manya Kahn's exercise class in New York twice a week, I can tell you the results are great!

The Aerobics Craze

Aerobic exercise is designed to increase your heart's efficiency by increasing its maximum rate of beats per minute—which will, in turn, and in time, cause it to pump more blood with fewer beats (or strokes) per minute when you are at rest. The results are achieved slowly, over a sustained program of exercise. The amount of aerobic exercise must be regulated, too, especially if you are out of condition. (If you've never run any great distance, it would be crazy to attempt a mile jog your first time out!)

The target zone. The maximum rate of the heart is approximately 220 beats per minute *minus* a number equal to your age. At forty, that would be 180. However you only want to increase the normal rate to a range of 70 to 80 percent of that number, the target zone (approximately 135 beats per minute, if you're forty) and only for the duration of the exercise, fifteen to thirty minutes, three to four times a week. A fit heart will return to its normal rate immediately afterward; the "normal" average falls between 60 and 100 (the lower the number at rest, the greater the indication of fitness).

Taking your pulse. To test your normal heart rate and to measure it after aerobic (or any) exercise, take your pulse; set a timer for thirty seconds and feel your pulse, at your wrist or by pressing your index fingers at the sides of your forehead. Count the number of beats in the thirty-second period. (If you hold your right palm up and back, you will probably be able to visually count the beats of the pulsing vein right at the wrist joint.) Multiply that number by two and you have your heart rate.

How to begin aerobics. Slowly, and after your doctor's okay. An aerobic exercise class is a good choice if you feel most comfortable with supervision (more on this later). You will increase the number of beats as you increase the level of exercise—the speed and the strength with which you do it. Remember, as when you diet, improvement is gradual.

AEROBIC CHOICES

· *Running.* On your own, start by walking for one minute, then running for one minute; repeat three times. Do this four times a week, every day if possible. At one-week intervals, add another minute of running to each one of walking:

Week 2: run 2, walk 1, run 2, walk 1, run 2, walk 1, etc.

Week 3: run 3, walk 1, run 3, walk 1, etc.

Week 4: run 4, walk 1, run 4, walk 1, etc.

When you can run for five sustained minutes, eliminate the walking step. Increase each run by one to three minutes, building to fifteen and up, if desired.

· *Swimming.* Many gyms and the Y offer an indoor swimming pool so that you can swim year-round. Start with as few as two laps back and forth; rest by holding on to the edge of the pool and kicking for one minute; then do two more laps. Then, as you feel able, increase the laps you swim between kicks until you reach five full minutes of laps. Build to fifteen and up, if desired.

· *Bicycling.* Start with one-mile stretches, walking the bike in between. Work up to three miles; add fractions of a mile each week, if that's your limit. Your goal is a fifteen-minute stretch at peak speed (don't take the sightseeing approach!). A very good alternate way to begin is on a stationary bike, your own or one at your gym. These can tell you how far you've gone and how fast; they have varying pressures to increase the exertion of your leg muscles. At home, bike while listening to the radio, if bored; at the gym, watch the odometer or read a book if that doesn't distract you from your pace.

· *Jumping Rope.* This exercise is more high-powered than the rest. Jump in ten-jump sets, catching your breath in between. Start with five sets a day, adding five sets a week until you reach fifty sets without stopping. Do this twice a day.

· *Cross-Country Skiing/Rowing.* Both are great, but not very practical for every day—unless your gym offers machines to simulate the actions of each. You can buy one or both of these machines to have at home, but each is space-consuming and can run as high as $2,000. On vacation, add these sports to your usual program if the season and place are right—or, if you wish, replace your program with them temporarily.

· *Walking.* See the following chart.

WALKING: THE AEROBIC EXERCISE FOR EVERYONE

Walking is the perfect exercise for almost everyone because it fits in so well with any kind of personal schedule. Done regularly, it will have an aerobic effect, but that's not all:

· Walking burns nearly 200 calories per half-hour if done vigorously.
· It improves your digestive system, and circulation in your legs (guarding against varicose veins), burns off fat, and reduces muscle fatigue as it strengthens and tones the legs.
· It brings more blood to the brain, easing mental tension, calming the nerves more effectively than a tranquilizer: hence the expression "I'm going for a walk to clear my head."

Optimally, you should walk a half-hour twice a day (back and forth from work or to the market or the movies). But start slowly: fifteen minutes at a brisk pace. Walk with determination and a purpose: to get where you're going as quickly, and eventually as effortlessly, as possible. Listen to your body to gauge your speed; challenge yourself a little more each day.

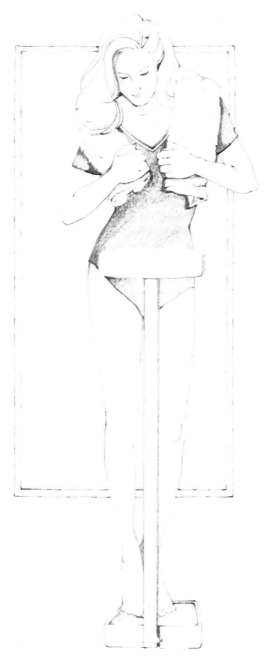

A GRAB BAG OF EXERCISE HINTS

Exercise the same time every time, especially when following an at-home program without supervision. If you can make your workout a daily habit, like brushing your hair, you'll stick with it.

- Wear comfortable clothing. Cotton shorts and a T-shirt with a good supportive bra underneath is great for any exercise, indoors or out: the cotton absorbs perspiration and allows your skin to breathe. Outdoors in cold weather, wear cotton underwear (long underwear is good) and layer on clothing that can be peeled off as you warm up: a jacket over a sweat shirt over a T-shirt instead of just one heavy jacket.
- Make every movement an exercise to encourage good tone and posture: a deep knee bend, keeping a straight back, when you pick up a box; a stretch from the waist when you bend or turn; a straight back with dropped, relaxed shoulders when you reach overhead for a book.
- Housework is a good exercise if you put your mind to it. The stretches and bends are excellent—and with a little concentrated effort, I can dust, vacuum, and make the bed in ten minutes.
- Exercise before you bathe/shower. The water acts as a relaxant to worked muscles, leaving you refreshed and freshened.
- An exercise mat makes exercising a little more pleasant—sometimes you just don't feel like plopping down on the carpet—and bare floors are hard. But you don't need any other gadgets or weight loss "aids."

PART III

Enhancing Your Natural Assets

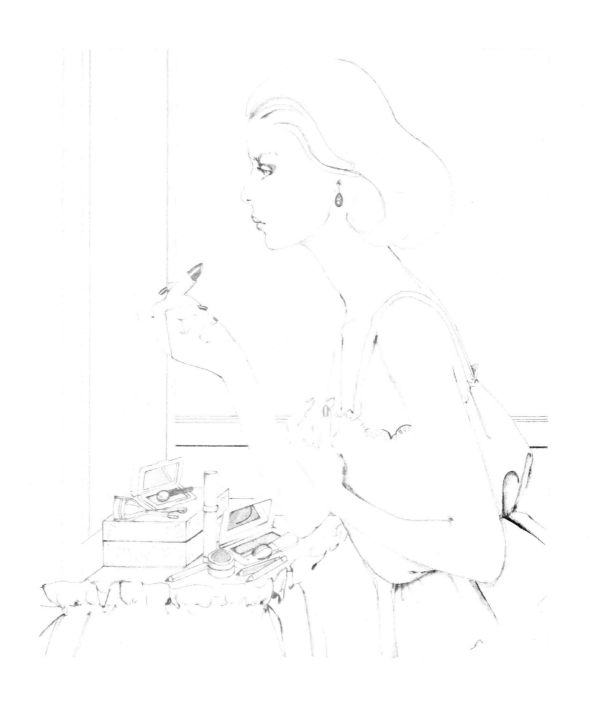

CHAPTER 7

Making the Most of Makeup

NINETEEN hundred and thirty-three was a landmark year for women—no, it wasn't the year we got the vote, it wasn't the year that we were released from corsets, but it *was* the year Max Factor introduced his pancake makeup; and the Western idea of beauty hasn't been the same since!

Gone forever was the original "natural look" that belonged to Grandma. At the time, that was gladly forsaken for the smooth, glowing surface Max's mixture provided. And for quite a time after that, too. In fact, it's taken us almost fifty years to question whether all that heavy makeup might be compromising our complexions. And the new "sheer" bases in creme and lotion form can also be damaging.

I don't believe there's any way to get around the fact that covering the skin every day, and over most of a lifetime, is going to have a progressively harmful effect: from lifeless skin to skin plagued by break-outs to skin whose lines ultimately deepen under the weight of the pigmented product.

Though equipped with this knowledge, force of habit keeps many of us at that jar every morning—applying foundation seems as important as brushing our teeth, and how could we ever give that up?

It's easier to minimize your use of makeup than you think. Convince yourself: Make your next vacation a vacation from makeup, too, or at least from foundation, powder and blush (face cosmetics). Give your complexion two solid weeks of thorough skin care—fourteen days to improve itself. Dermabrase every day if your skin tolerates it well (remember that very fair, sensitive skin may not: in that case try every other day, or only once a week, always with very light pressure). You'll be pleased with the results.

When you return home, make the most of your eye makeup, as I do, use lipstick, and some blush if you need it for color or shine; leave out the rest.

I prefer a light touch when it comes to makeup—a bright lipstick, a few strokes of mascara, a brush of blush.

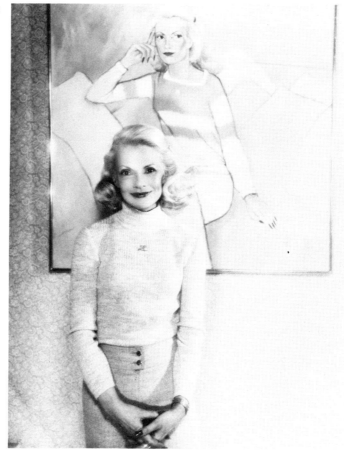

With minimizing your use of cosmetics in mind, I offer you the following thoughts and ideas on selective makeup—makeup chosen only as you need it, used in the most discriminating way.

THE ART OF MAKEUP

I believe that the best use of makeup results in the application you don't see—people should compliment you on how well you're looking, not on the fabulous color of your lipstick. To accomplish this, using a minimum of makeup is a must—if you keep using a lot, there's no way to avoid looking painted. (Most men, incidentally, do not like to see the hard look that comes from wearing heavy or very obvious makeup; they think of it not only as intimidating, but vulgar as well.)

Of course, we each have a different concept of what the minimum is. Makeup is one reflection of your personal style. Women who don't fuss over their hair or clothes rarely spend hours on their makeup; those who insist on being impeccably groomed at all times wouldn't get the mail without first putting on lipstick. But if you're in the middle, and like to use makeup to your best advantage, you think in terms of its appropriateness to the occasion.

Every woman has more than one facet to her personality, and a different degree of makeup is needed for each. The jogger does not think of including foundation, blusher or even lipstick (though a protective lip cream is in order) in her "warm-up." But when the businesswoman in her surfaces, a light, careful makeup that considers her eyes, lips and cheeks is on her list; but she keeps it simple because daylight intensifies makeup. And when she's up for a night on the town, she might take makeup a little further—glossier lips and heavily mascara'ed eyes to compensate for the color-draining lighting of the usual night spots.

The art of makeup means suiting it to the event and to your moods, not trying to make a statement with your face—that is the key to looking like yourself at all times, and at all times your best self. Once you achieve this, you have mastered makeup. Experimenting, at home and in stores, and learning the intricacies of your face, is the only way to do it—every woman's face is unique and no book can tell each individual what, specifically, to do. Ignoring this uniqueness is the fault of most makeup books and the reason that I seek only to guide you with general impressions that can really be applied to all.

ON SELECTION

I'm certain that I won't be able to persuade all of you to abandon your foundation, no matter how aging I say it is—especially if you feel that you need it for coverage. Select only the sheerest, lightest water-based product that is easily applied. Creme and thick liquids coat the skin, sink into lines and crack as you make a facial expression. Do check the foundation on your face before you buy: many water-based ones are not as thin as they should be. The color should approximate your best skin tone, whether it be ivory, light rose, coffee or deep brown. Be careful about using the beige shades: the yellow pigments will draw attention to a sallow tone, particularly under bright fluorescent lights.

Avoid face powders. To get rid of shine, don't layer on powder—oils will cause it to cake. Remove the oils instead. Place a tissue over the area(s) and hold it firmly in place. Run a finger of the other hand back and forth across the tissue (don't allow the tissue itself to move). It will absorb the oils. For very oily skin, it's better to cleanse the face and get a clean start with new makeup.

You can use a light creme or a powder blush unless you find that the pigments are clogging the pores. I often prefer to blend the color from my lipstick with my moisturizer to have a custom-made blush—I achieve a harmonious shade and I know that the blush is moisturizing as I wear it. Lipstick—I see a return to the indelible type for long-lasting color; it stays on all day, shined by gloss as needed. Pencils define the lip line, and improve every smile.

The eyes—select shadows in neutral colors—waves of green, blue, purple are out. Mascara, yes; false eyelashes, no. Eyeliner that's smoky, not hard line, to define the lashes.

Makeup formats—gels, cremes, powders, cakes—are a matter of personal preference, as long as your complexions's characteristics are considered first. For instance, cremes will not last well on oily skin; they can melt off with excess oil secretions and can worsen clogged pores and break-outs. Try powder blush and shadows—but to achieve a more natural and lasting look, apply them wet: use a moistened cotton ball to apply blush, a wet blush or moistened cotton swab for shadows and hard-to-reach areas. You will have greater control over intensity and placement. On the other hand, dry skin that has been properly moisturized might comfortably "hold" powders applied dry or wet, though you might prefer the more malleable cremes.

Buy only what you'll use in short order. Makeup freshness is a must for the most successful application.

ON COLOR

The makeup industry tries to mirror changes in the fashion world—new styles and shades every season. That's fine for those who let fashion dictate to them, but I don't believe in adapting your face to every fad any more than you should your wardrobe. Inventing and promoting bizarre colors and exaggerated looks (triple-shade eye shadowing and the like) is not my approach—it is why I have stayed put in skin care. I believe in looking for the truest shades, the ones that enhance and define, not the ones you paint on (those faces would look better hanging at the Museum of Modern Art!). After all, the only reason to wear makeup (and this escapes so many women who rush out to buy gold glitter and mocha lipstick at the drop of an ad) is to enhance your features. Finding shades that add to your beauty is hard enough; switching them successfully four times a year is an impossibility, and as silly a concept as changing your hair color or entirely replacing your wardrobe every fashion season.

Colors: subtle neutrals, muted shades, the spectrum of pales, but not the bold, blaring white-lip, black-eye look (not *those* neutrals), not the glaring greens and blues, oranges and red blue-reds. Harmony between eye/cheek/lip color (and nails, too, if polished) is makeup at its best. These most expressive features are best enhanced when considered in relation to each other. Colors should be from the same palette—rose/mauve; bronze/spice; peach/tawn; burgundy/berry. Start lightly; soften colors with a few drops of moisturizer in your palm before stroking on; always think of flattering your complexion.

ON APPLICATION

Foremost is preparing the skin. For maximum makeup performance, the skin must be scrupulously clean and moisturized. Even if you followed the seven-minute routine right before bed, the next morning calls for it again: a night's worth of dead skin cells and oil secretions needs to be washed away.

Prepare your surroundings. Have everything handy, including a good mirror: *clean* (dust and pollutants collect on the surface every day) and *large* (a compact-sized mirror won't do the trick). A double vanity mirror or medicine chest doors that swing out are wonderful for checking applications at all angles.

Lighting is crucial. More makeup mistakes are due to incorrect lighting than any other cause. If you'll be outdoors primarily, make up at a table placed at a window. Bright bathroom lights simulate those at the office. Lighted mirrors aren't always reliable; you'll have to check on arrival at the office. Save pink bulbs for romantic evenings. Dim lights are great in all other rooms, but for the bath, get all the white wattage your fixture can hold.

A "light hand" is in order—and most women, once they learn of the advantages, *do* wear less makeup. The women who work in my office are a perfect example. When they are first employed, they often seem heavy-handed in applying their makeup, to compensate for lifeless skin. But as they are introduced to my simple skin-care system, they need less and less, and consequently wear less and less. You see, it's not just the need for makeup that's bad, it's the incongruous fact that, though designed to make you look better, makeup very often merely draws attention to less than flawless skin. (And if your skin is flawless, why wear any?)

Apply only the thinnest veil of foundation with a damp sponge; pat over hard-to-cover areas with a second touch-up, rather than smearing on one heavy coat right from the bottle.

Blush deepens the rose of your cheeks; apply first in the center, the "apples" of your cheeks, then bring it up and out gradually along the cheekbones until it fades into the natural tone of your skin, giving you that look of vitality, all over if you like—across the forehead and temples, the bridge of the nose, the browbones of the upper eyelids.

Lipstick can be more vibrant: pencil to define, color to fill in, gloss for the shiny finish if needed. A brush gives added control for narrow corners.

FOR THE EYES

I love eye makeup—it can make such a difference. In fact, it's often the only makeup I use, except for gala occasions.

Press a tissue over each lid to absorb any moisture that could cause creasing, smudges. Then apply shadow –selected to enhance the eye, not match its color. Before you try the latest three-color shadow trick, ask yourself if wearing any "color" is really right for you. I like only a hint of blush or tawn across the lid, well blended, with no telltale demarcation. Next, a neutral brown on the natural crease beneath the browbone adds depth and warmth to the eyes.

One eye makeup tool you probably don't yet think of as an essential: the eyelash curler. Use it on clean unmade-up lashes and you can throw

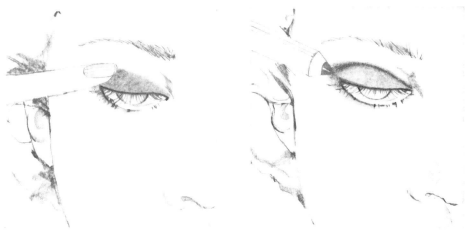

Applying shadow.   *Adding depth.*

Curling lashes.   *Intensifying with mascara.*

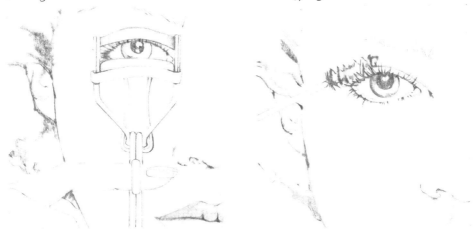

away your false lashes (I have!). After making certain the rubber strip is clean and intact, press the curler down at the roots and hold for a count of five. Slowly release the curler and dab the tips of your lashes with moisturizer or night creme for conditioning and shine.

If your lashes are dark or dyed, you may not need mascara. But if you want them to appear thicker or darker, use black in either wand or cake form. First roll the brush along the topside of upper lashes to distribute color evenly; next, the underside, and finally, holding the wand vertically, brush across the lower lashes. Define further by dotting at the roots with an eyebrow pencil for a more natural look.

If you're uncertain about your "look," a makeup artist can clue you in to something you may have neglected, an asset you haven't played to full advantage. He/she can tell you if you should sweep blush across your cheeks or center it only on the "apples." But don't succumb to even the most reknowned wizard if he or she wants to turn your face into a canvas subject to his or her whims and perhaps folly (demonstrators at makeup counters are notorious for this). Remember, you get what you pay for: pass up the "free" make-over for a private session with a professional.

MAKEUP AS CORRECTION

Many women with close-set eyes make them appear wider apart by concentrating mascara and liner at the outer corners of the eyelids—that's enhancement. I don't feel that my mouth is my best feature, so I define my lips with a pencil—that's enhancement, too. I used to shade my nose to make it look thinner (I was so used to seeing perfect noses around me that I began wondering about my own)—that's correction.

I stopped the brown shading one day when I realized that a thin nose would only make my mouth look too wide. All your features have to work together; "fixing" one can work against all the others. Ask yourself if it's really your nose that's keeping you from looking great. Or is it that you need to revamp your makeup completely?

You can see that shading is a tricky business. It's magic if you're adept, but black magic if you're not—the kind that's dangerous. The major drawback is that the brown shadings are noticeable everywhere but the eyes, where natural creases are heightened. Along the lower outline of the cheekbones, the straight sides of the nose, the planes of the jawline—these are difficult to shade well. It takes a lot of work, a lot of practice to get it right, and above all, instruction by a professional to show you where and how you can make the most difference.

AS YOUR FACE CHANGES

It's vital to look at yourself—and reevaluate your makeup needs —as you enter different periods in your life. Your body doesn't stay the same, and neither do your features. You must be aware of these changes because, if you wear makeup, your application techniques must change as well.

A woman's face becomes more defined with time:

The cheekbones often become more prominent, and blusher will have to be adjusted to emphasize the sweep of bone.

Fine lines may appear above the upper lip, and using a pencil to outline the lips before applying color will be needed to prevent "bleeding."

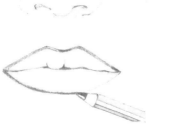
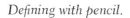
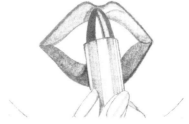

Defining with pencil.   *Adding color.*

The eyelids change, too, giving eyes more depth and interest, and less need for makeup. Avoid the busy-ness of smudged eyeshadow, of complicated applications of color, of dabbing on concealer to hide shadows or puffiness (the creme will merely seep into the lines and exaggerate them).

Using less makeup in general and choosing clear, bright colors instead of murky tones that pale the skin further keep you looking fresh and vibrant. Experiment as always, and judge with objectivity.

That sounds easy, but I found out just how difficult it can be, especially when being objective neccesitates *changing*. I loved and habitually wore a dark-brick lipstick—I thought the color was wonderful. Well, after a time, my friends, one by one, started hinting that I should try a new color. No, no, I insisted. It had taken me a long time to find this one, and I was sticking to it.

Leave it to my manicurist to outsmart me! I was having my nails done—it was mid-spring—and she suggested I try a pale-pink polish for summer months (naturally the brick color had been on my nails all this time, too). Before I could answer, she had taken matters into her own hands and was applying the pink shade. Then she added, "Of course, you can't keep wearing that brown on your lips—the two colors clash. You'll have to change your lipstick." I immediately went in search of a complementing color, found it, used it—and started receiving all sorts of compliments! My look had changed fantastically. The moral: Listen to the suggestions of those around you, especially if they come from someone (your husband, one of your kids) who rarely says anything— it'll be doubly important. Listen, and you'll be surprised with the results.

Your makeup may not be the only thing lagging behind. You can get so used to a set image of yourself that you fight against changing it —a completely "normal" reaction: we all love a rut, it's comfy and cozy, even if it's not very exciting. It could be your clothes, even your hairstyle. I have a friend who is very tailored in her daytime approach: she always wears a smart suit, her makeup and nails are always impeccable, her hair is always set in a straight, simple style with a flip at the ends, every strand just so (the kind of style that would prompt a stranger to say to her, "wake up—we're in the eighties now!") Well, one day, we were meeting for lunch and the weather was very rainy and windy. My friend's perfect hair was tousled about her head by the time she reached our destination—a wreck, in her opinion. But to everyone in the restaurant, she looked vivacious and sexy. I pleaded with her to have her hairdresser bring this haphazard quality to her hair the next time he styled it. She protested at first, complaining that it was really a mess, but she finally agreed to ask her stylist's opinion. He concurred happily with me and the other diners, and her hair now has a new aliveness, though still with graceful ease.

As all women get older—and I don't mean old age, I mean, as we approach our forties, even our thirties—we tend to forget about experimenting with makeup, fashion, hairstyles, the fun things we used to try out in the privacy of our dressing room (if they don't work out, no one else has to know). Don't retire your beauty to the shelf before its time. You can find new vitality if you look for it.

BEAUTY ON THE GO

At the office, or after dinner, or even 30,000 feet in the air—these are some of the times you might need to touch up your makeup. Cosmetics wear off, and not always evenly; they smudge, too, especially around the eyes. Lipstick can be quickly reapplied, a wet swab can whisk away smears under the eyes. But putting another layer of foundation or even blush on skin that still has traces of old makeup—well, it's like putting on perfume when you really should shower.

Quick cleansing, avoiding the eye area (leaving mascara *et al* intact) and reapplying face basics are easy when you have a cosmetics case with portables: mini-sizes of cleanser and moisturizer. (Always look for gifts-with-purchase specials from your favorite manufacturers.) Also add to your portable perk-up kit the following little niceties that repair potentially disastrous mishaps:

- emery board
- nail polish, if used
- hand and body lotion
- hairbrush
- perfume or cologne
- eye drops
- lint brush
- needle and thread
- cotton swabs
- spare hose
- toothbrush (more effective than covering up with mouthwash; can be done as quickly, and *without* paste)
- a magnifying mirror to make up for not having a large one

ON REMOVING MAKEUP

Just a note to remind you that taking makeup *off* is of more value to your skin than putting it on. For the best results, take a look at page 48.

CHAPTER 8

New Perspectives: Cautions for Cosmetic Surgery

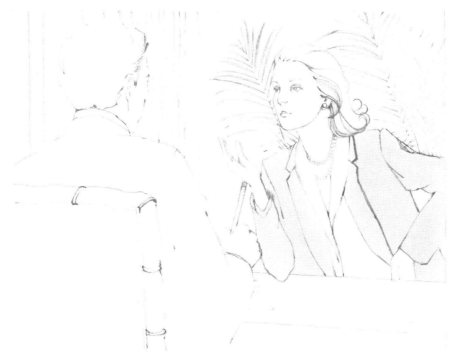

A consultation with a surgeon.

THE advances that have taken place in the field of plastic surgery are phenomenal. Though we are often most intrigued by the wonders of cosmetic surgery, the truly astounding strides are the ones made in the area of reconstruction, to correct birth defects and repair damage.

One of these wonder stories was told to me by a Mrs. America, the year I helped judge the contest. This beautiful lady recounted a tragic car accident ten years earlier; her face was so badly damaged that it had to be totally reconstructed (so much so that she hardly resembled her old photographs, so well that she entered the contest and won the year after her last operation). The miracle is that her life was saved, that this kind of surgery is possible—it's no wonder that women look to plastic surgery as a way to a new identity, a new beginning. But I can tell you that the Mrs. America I speak of would have gladly passed up the title to have avoided the ordeal she endured.

Yes, the day has come when we can change everything: the nose, the chin, the ears. But this all has to be put back into perspective. These techniques can be life-saving; but used as casually as mascara, we can be in for a great deal of trouble.

We've certainly demystified the facelift—it's no longer the well-guarded secret it was thirty years ago. But it's still not like a visit to the hairdresser's, as many magazine articles would have us believe. Women are led to draw unrealistic expectations of what the surgery can do for them, and they have too little conception of what it really involves.

> ## ELECTIVE SURGERY MEANS YOU WANT IT, NOT THAT YOU NEED IT

If you are seriously considering surgery for purely cosmetic reasons (personal beautification), think it out fully. I want you to put yourself through a very simple test to see just how serious you are; read this entire chapter. Here is a frank discussion of the details you don't always read about—not just the descriptions of the different operations (your surgeon will inform you in more detail—*listening* to him is test number 2), but also the wrong reasons for electing surgery and the most common false expectations you're likely to have. There is also the anxiety and the physical discomfort to consider. I'm not sure I could go through all that trauma—could you?

Filling in the Gaps—Some Startling Facts You May Not Have Known

1. *The results of a facelift are by no means permanent.* Often they hardly qualify as long-lasting. Because aging occurs at different rates, it is hard to predict how long it will be before you once again look the way you did prior to surgery. But aging is inevitable: the operation can

turn the clock back a bit, but can't turn it off, can't stop body processes in any way.

Your skin will start slackening right away, at its previous rate. As a very general rule that means a second lift can be done in five to eight years (of course, it is not mandatory to have another). But there are many exceptions—the effects may last from two years to fifteen. It all depends on your skin's elasticity, the factor that determines skin's ability to contract after it is stretched (in speaking, eating, frowning) and to resist sagging into creases and folds. To judge your elasticity factor, compare the look of your skin to that of people your age—if it has stood up well, it has greater elasticity. If, on the other hand, you feel you need a lift early in life, say before forty, your skin has little elasticity and you will need another lift sooner.

A second lift should be just a series of tucks because there is the increased danger of pulling skin too tight, of straining its elasticity and compromising its blood supply: skin will take on a dull, stretched look. Remember: there's no limit to how many lifts you can have, but there is a limit to how much you can accomplish each successive time.

2. *Most operations are performed under* LOCAL *anesthesia.* There are sound reasons for this—less swelling and bruising—but it can be traumatic. You won't feel any physical pain until the local wears off, but you will be awake, aware of the doctors, the instruments, the medical talk and the operating room in all its splendor. Injections are made directly to the areas being operated on: the cheeks, the eyelids. . . . It can be quite distressing just to imagine.

3. *For up to three weeks afterward you will look worse.* The Catch-22 of cosmetic surgery is that it doesn't always improve your looks, at least at first. And some aftereffects can last a long time.

Bruises (black-and-blue marks that are the normal result of bleeding under the skin) are the first things you see, even before bandages are removed. Those resulting from eye or nose surgery can last up to ten days—from a lift, up to three weeks. Swelling can cause the whole face to blow up or one eye to look larger than the other.

Bandages cover the stitches that go around the ears after a facelift, along the lower lashlines and across the upper lid creases after an eye "lift," under the chin after the neck "lift." Often the bandages form a turban and are left in place for up to a week, depending on how well you heal.

Scars will result anywhere an incision has been made. Usually they are located within natural curves and creases for minimal detection and will fade to thin white lines if you heal well (if too much skin has been removed, scars may not heal as well). Figure out your healing potential by examining your body. Do you have noticeable scars from any past cuts or wounds? Are old vaccination marks inconspicuous?

4. *There are risks.* The notion of having early-morning surgery at the doctor's office and feeling rested enough to cook dinner is quite unlikely. (You are always advised to rest at least one day afterward with your head elevated.) Particularly for the full lift, it's important to have the security of a hospital. Of course, the percentages are in favor of no complications, but what a comfort to know that all emergency equipment is available—when complications happen to you, who cares about the percentages anyway?

There is a risk of complications with any surgical procedure. For facelifts, they can include: excessive bleeding and bruising, infection and muscle weakness (which can account for one eye appearing larger than the other). Fortunately, they can all be corrected by the surgeon, with little chance of permanent damage. In extreme cases, the sutures will have to be opened.

5. *Discomfort exists.* There's no question about it. Think of how uncomfortable a paper cut is, then try convincing yourself that a major incision won't bother you—it can't be done.

In addition, you may experience numbness or a loss of sensitivity at the back of the neck, around the ears, anywhere. The eyes can be irritated by the swelling; the skin, from the bandages (much more so after body-contouring surgery).

6. *No refunds, no exchanges.* If you buy new makeup and decide you don't need it by the time you get home, chances are the store will refund your money when you return it the next day. If you don't like your facelift . . . well, you'd better look again. Unless there has been gross negligence on the part of the surgeon (like the famous case of the tummy tuck that resulted in the navel being placed six inches to the left—or was it to the right?), what you see is . . . You know the rest.

And financially, the surgery is expensive. In New York, a facelift can run between $3,000 to $6,000, before the hospital costs are added on! (Elective surgery fees are usually higher than non-emergency services.) A higher fee is *not* necessarily a confirmation of a surgeon's expertise—he may simply be taking advantage of the public's misconception that if it costs more it must be better.

7. *We make no guarantees.* Those are the words of a plastic surgeon.

Facts on Procedures

Here is a run-down of the most frequently performed operations. These are all average estimates of operating time, healing time and the like and can vary depending on individual characteristics and complications. Put simply: it won't get any better than this.

THE FACE-SAVING PROCEDURES FOR TURNING BACK THE CLOCK

THE FACELIFT:
- *removes* sagging folds of skin around the contours of the face
- *operating time:* two to five hours depending on the extent of the "redraping"
- *incisions:* surround each ear (if they cut across the scalp within the hairline, a thin strip of hair will be shaved, but as it is not too close to the hairline, its loss shouldn't be apparent)
- *stitches:* some are removed within a week, the rest before the end of the second week
- *healing:* three weeks for swelling to go down and taut feeling to ease, bruises to fade, longer for pink scars to turn white
   The drawbacks:
- a facelift will not remove those deep, fine lines that are etched into the skin, often by sun exposure. Facelifts lift off excess folds of skin, not surface lines which have to do with its texture, not its volume. Don't mislead yourself into having false hopes by looking into the mirror and pulling skin back with your hands at the center of the cheeks or at the temples. The tucks are made behind the ears and within the hairline. Reposition your hands—are the projected results as good?
- a loss of sensitivity can last months—in the sun you won't even know when you're hot or burning
- the lengthy healing period
- blood clots—these can disappear spontaneously or be removed, but in rare instances sutures will have to be opened to do so
- incisions won't heal correctly and face will take on a masklike look if the skin is pulled too tightly. There is an increased danger of this with subsequent lifts, when there is a tendency on the part of the surgeon to overcorrect

- on a man's skin: shaving will have to be adjusted. Sideburns move up and the beard extends behind the ears if the lift is a good one

THE NECKLIFT OR "TURKEY GOBBLER-ECTOMY"
- *improves* jaw and neck line when performed in conjunction with a facelift. Some surgeons will correct this area by itself, using a procedure that sutures the new lines around the ear lobes
- *operating time:* twenty minutes to one hour
- *incisions:* made in the crease under the chin
- *stitches:* removed as with the facelift
- *healing:* bruises and swelling fade in a week
    The drawbacks:
- all those for the facelift

THE EYELID LIFT-AND-TUCK:
- *removes* the fatty tissue that collects in the lower lids and the folds of the upper lid. Often the eyes are done years before a facelift. Conversely, most surgeons recommend you have the eyes done when you have a lift if they haven't been done before, or if there is the slightest need, because they will look worse after other parts of the face have been corrected. Heredity can be a major factor causing a need for this surgery as early as age twenty and for health reasons if the drooping lids obscure the vision
- *operating time:* one to two hours; however extreme cases can take up to three and a half hours
- *incisions:* on the upper lid, made across the natural crease; on the lower lid, made under the lashline
- *stitches:* removed after three days
- *healing:* one to two weeks for swelling and bruises to fade
    The drawbacks:
- all those for the facelift
- eyelids can jut out from the eyes for a few weeks following surgery because of muscle weakness
- eyelids may not perfectly match each other after surgery: one eye may look more open than the other
- increased chance of eye irritation/infection
- if too much skin is removed, you may not be able to close lids tightly, can lose reflex action that shuts out dust, etc.

THE CORRECTION PROCEDURES TO
GRACE YOU AS NATURE NEVER DID

THE NOSE JOB:
- *changes* the contours of your nose
- *operating time:* one to two hours depending upon whether a deviated septum is corrected as well
- *incisions:* all made within the nose
- *stitches:* within nostrils if their shape has been changed; otherwise only a splint, removed from two to seven days afterward
- *healing:* one week for swelling and bruises around eyes and nose, but it takes six to twelve months for the nose to take its final shape

The drawbacks:
- loss of individuality. In my acting and modeling days, a few people remarked that my nose was wide and would photograph better after plastic surgery. This, of course, led me to my father's office as a regular patient for a consultation. He explained that a narrower nose would only upset the balance of my face and detract from a certain elfin personality that my own "imperfect" but unique nose contributed. Other surgeons weren't as honest or as skilled. Many doled out one of a handful of standard noses—you could tell by the nose who had done the surgery. Thankfully, today's techniques are more sophisticated. A surgeon can draw new contours on your nose during your consultation to help you see what improvements can be made. (Any surgeon worth his weight in scalpels will tell you that you have to be at least fifteen or sixteen before having a nose job; for girls, waiting until menstruation starts is a must—facial bone growth ceases after that.)
- you will have to breathe through your mouth for a few days while packing fills your nostrils
- expect one or two days of bleeding after surgery
- numbness, especially at the tip of the nose, can last for weeks

NOTE: A new nose won't turn a plain Jane into a raving beauty. Makeup techniques can do more. I suggest a real fling: go to a makeup artist—not one at a cosmetics counter whose chief interest is in getting you to buy all the products he/she applies—but one who works on a consultation basis. Since individual features are in vogue, large noses especially, ask about turning your "flaw" into an asset.

THE EAR TUCK:
- *pins* back protruding ears. Clark Gable may have made a fortune with

his, but you may not be so lucky. For emotional well-being, especially for that of a youngster (after the age of five is usually okay), this may be the most justifiable of all cosmetic procedures, coming closest to repairing a disfigurement. It is usually performed under general anesthesia in the case of a child

- *operating time:* one to two hours
- *incisions:* all behind the ears
- *stitches:* removed after one week
- *healing:* swelling and bruises around ear fade after one week
  The drawbacks:
- some throbbing lasting a day or more
- a turban of bandages (like that of the facelift) in place for up to a week; a knit band will be needed when you sleep, for up to two months

THE ENDOWMENTS FROM THE SILICONE BANK

NOTE: the use of silicone injections is now, luckily, restricted. They were used everywhere (furrows, acne pits, breasts) and with disastrous results. Loose silicone travels (from cheekbones to jowls—the chipmunk effect), infiltrates surrounding tissue (and you can't withdraw it), migrates (from the breasts to the liver!). The following procedures involve silicone *implants:* solution sealed into sacs.

CHIN AUGMENTATION:
- *implants* an addition directly on the bone to increase a weak chin
- *operating time:* thirty minutes
- *incision:* through the lower lip or under the chin
- *stitches:* removed after one week
- *healing:* swelling and bruises lighten in one week
  The drawbacks:
- you are living with an implant that can become damaged in an accident; you must exercise extreme caution
- the body may have an unpredictable adverse reaction to the artificial material you've introduced
- all the complications of surgery

BREAST AUGMENTATION:
implants add dimension directly beneath natural breast tissues

- *operating time*: about two hours; can be performed under a general anesthetic if you wish
- *incisions*: can vary from woman to woman, depending on individual figures. This should be an important point in your discussion with your doctor
- *stitches*: removed within a week, protected by a bra-type bandage
- *healing*: swelling and bruising decreasing within two weeks, but no exercise permitted during this time. A decrease in sensitivity can last one month or longer

  The drawbacks:
- same as for the chin augmentation
- there is a permanent scar outlining the bottom of the areola, though it will fade to a white line
- sensitivity can be lost for months, but should return

BREAST RECONSTRUCTION AFTER A MASTECTOMY

Women bear a double cross when breast cancer strikes. First, naturally, they must cope with the disease; and second, sometimes with even more difficulty, they must face the loss of so visible a part of the body. For those who wish to consider breast reconstruction, you should know that it is often possible, either within a week of the surgery or any time after three months later. Though it is a far more complicated procedure than breast augmentation, it does involve implants that, to date, have not been shown to cause a repeat of cancer, nor does their positioning interfere with its detection.

The drawbacks include the emotional trauma of facing more surgery and, as with all cosmetic surgery, there aren't any guarantees that you will look as you used to—but photos will help you see the difference the technique can make. You will have to weigh all these factors to decide what is best for you.

THE BODY TUCKS

BREAST REDUCTION:
- *corrects* the size of pendulous breasts that can cause physical damage: back problems, pressure that results in bad posture, slumping shoulders and ridges, even poor sleeping habits

- *operating time:* three to five hours, under a general anesthesia
- *incisions:* depend largely on the size of the breasts and the amount of reconstruction needed for the desired shape. Your doctor should be able to show you where scars will be noticeable, and where they will fade to a thin, white line
- *stitches:* removed within two weeks, protected by a bra-type bandage
- *healing:* same as for breast augmentation

The drawbacks:
- permanent decrease in sensitivity may occur, primarily around the nipples
- breast feeding will almost certainly be impossible
- scars may not heal well if too much skin is removed

NOTE: Before taking so serious a course of action, visit an experienced corsetière who will properly measure you and outfit you with bras that offer the most comfort and support. Very often the physical problems mentioned above can happen to anyone (regardless of breast size) who does not wear the correct, supportive bra.

BODY CONTOURING:
- *trims* the body of excess skin and fat through surgery on the tummy, the hips, the buttocks, the legs and/or the arms (some women have had entire bodies done; others have even had fanny implants for a rounder derrière!)
- *operating time:* lengthy and very complicated
- *incisions:* very long, leaving very visible permanent scars (nowhere to conceal them on the length of a leg)
- *stitches:* exceedingly numerous, complicated bandages
- *healing:* very long

The drawbacks:

Many. These are major operations (the specifics about each will vary) and therefore all the risks of major surgery are attached to them, most importantly the loss of sensitivity to large parts of the body. To me, these procedures are even more awesome than the thought of having one's face operated on, and potentially more dangerous.

NOTE: because of the length of the scars, you probably won't be in a bathing suit too frequently. Since revealing clothes will be restricted anyway, why not learn to wear clothes that flatter your present shape as you diet faithfully—and forget about having fat surgically removed.

Sound Reasoning

There are as many wrong reasons to have cosmetic surgery as there are good ones. How reasonable does your reasoning sound?

WHY? You feel that your looks are holding you back, are standing in the way of your merits. A retailing executive I know had the surgery and his career climbed—success as easily attributed to the self-confidence he recaptured as to the youthful appearance he regained.

WHY NOT? You hope Burt Reynolds will knock down your door or you'll look like Candy Bergen—expectations as unrealistic as thinking a facelift will bring back the husband who left you (he probably didn't leave because of *your* wrinkles).

WHY? You no longer like what you see in the mirror and your facial contours have started adversely affecting your personality. A real desire to improve yourself, for yourself—you can usually fool everyone else with a deft makeup application.

WHY NOT? You have the urge for a change. If that's how you feel, it's safer and cheaper to buy yourself a whole new wardrobe—even to have it selected for you! Women are rarely satisfied when they have surgery for the wrong reasons and that can lead to disaster: when the facelift doesn't bring anticipated results, they try the ears, the nose . . . Trouble ahead!

WHY? You have a real need, at any age. Even a twenty-seven-year-old can have skin with such poor elasticity that she looks years older. (This of course is still rare.) And don't have surgery just because you feel that you've gotten to "that age."

WHY NOT? As a cure-all for emotional distress. My father often told me that he had to play part doctor, part psychiatrist at every consultation to determine how real the problem was. (Visually, it's easy for a trained professional to tell, but advising the surgery for cosmetic reasons may not cure the real ill if the problem is emotional.) His answer for one patient was to wear higher heels to give her the long, lanky look she wanted. Her original idea, to have her chin done, would never have accomplished that! (Most well-adjusted women are so at home with themselves at every age that cosmetic surgery is never more than a fleeting thought—like owning the Hope diamond.)

If you think that the only thing standing between you and a life of contentment is breast augmentation, you're misleading yourself. The real shame here is that if you're that determined you'll ignore sound medical advice to the contrary and go elsewhere—and you'll always be able to find a doctor willing (do not read: ethical) to do the surgery. Be honest with yourself, or you'll be back at a reputable surgeon's office six months later, asking him to undo the damage.

The Consultation

If the problem is real and the solution is clear, you'll want the most capable doctor available. Start by asking your family doctor, your dermatologist, satisfied friends; do a little discreet inquiring after snipped-and-tucked socialites in your area. Never follow up on an advertisement in a newspaper—I shudder when I think of what my father would have to say about that practice!

Overlook the endorsements or other mention of surgeons in your favorite magazines—today all that means is a good public-relations agent. Don't ask the surgeon for case histories—it's a snap for a doctor to pull out three beautiful "after shots" from the thousands of operations he's performed. You want living proof you've discovered on your own. Find three friends or acquaintances or friends of friends who have had successful surgery performed by the same doctor (hopefully a surgeon recommended by your GP or dermatologist). Three. One is not enough; the patient could have the ideal requirements: skin that adapts well to surgery, and heals well, too. Two is still iffy. You want three—I never said this part was easy, but it's your face, isn't it?

Your subjects must look natural, as though they just came back from a marvelous vacation. The best kudo you can give a surgeon is that his patient still looks like herself. That's what you want for yourself, too.

When you set up a consultation with the surgeon, carefully evaluate your needs; consider each part of your face: the forehead, the cheeks, the eyes, the jawline, the neck. You want the finished results to be harmonious.

If the surgeon advises you not to elect surgery at the present time, *stop*. On the way home, count your blessings and buy yourself something extravagant.

If he agrees with you, treat yourself to a second opinion—perhaps the wisest money you'll ever spend. Clearly explain to the second doctor that you want only a consultation, that the surgery would be done by the first surgeon you saw, if you decide on it, to assure the most honest evaluation.

If both doctors agree with you, review the procedure, the after-effects, the potential complications. Think long and hard. Make a decision you can stick with, even if your answer is to wait a full year and then to reevaluate. With cosmetic surgery, there's no turning back.

Pre-Op . . . Post-Op

Before the surgery:
· lose all the weight you can. You want skin to be as loose as possible so that as much as is feasibly possible can be removed. This is true for any kind of surgery (before a gallbladder removal, for example) to achieve the neatest incision, the thinnest scars. Losing weight will also help reduce needed tucks in the fat fold of the neck
· lead a simple lifestyle prior to the surgery. Cut out all alcohol, all medication (unless your doctor suggests otherwise), even aspirin, as these can cause greater swelling, bleeding and bruising
· if you color your hair, have it done a week before surgery. Wash it the night before (you'll usually do this in the hospital, as check-in is the day before)
· find out about a hairdresser who has worked with postoperative patients from your doctor—he can best see to your post-op hair needs. If you want to keep your surgery a secret, make sure your hairdresser is discreet—he'll be the second to know as soon as he sees the scars during your next appointment
· follow all your surgeon's specific instructions. Ask questions

After surgery:
· it's essential to reevaluate your skin care and makeup needs so that you don't start making the same mistakes that helped age the skin in the first place
· stay out of the sun completely for six weeks. After that time, use a sunblock—always. The loss of sensitivity will keep you from knowing when the sun is too hot; the sun's rays can also redden healing scars. Limit exposure at all costs; skin is more vulnerable now than ever
· you'll have to wait three weeks at least to color your hair; two at least before you can use makeup

- follow all your doctor's instructions, especially those concerning limits on physical activity and tips for proper healing

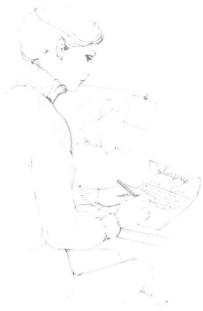

A Final Word . . .

At the beginning of this chapter I said that a good indication of your desire would be the ability to get through these pages. So you've made it. Well, I'd like to leave you with one other anti-cosmetic surgery argument if you're still considering a change, if you're still debating.

I want you to believe, as I do, that it is important for women to start thinking more positively about themselves by putting less emphasis on the external. At the beginning of what was to be a spectacular career—though she didn't know it then—Sophia Loren refused to change her Roman nose. Today, past the age of forty, she is still considered one of the most beautiful women in the world. It's about time we all began to follow this lovely lady's lead.

Equally important is not letting the current preoccupation with looking twenty forever make anyone over the age of twenty-five start worrying about her looks, and certainly not letting it lead her to thoughts of surgical solutions. Yes, concentrate on looking *better*, but remember that's not a synonym for "younger." It merely means looking your loveliest at every age.

CHAPTER 9

Irma's Always Asked ...

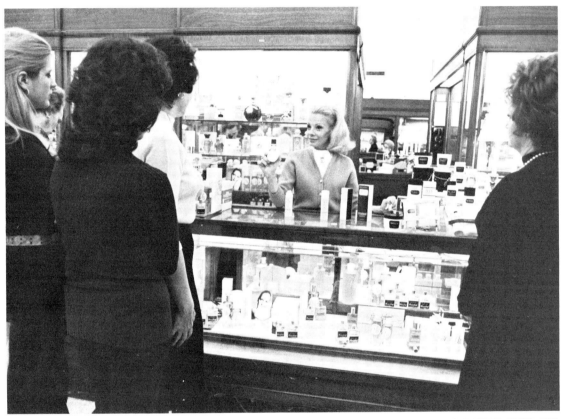

FOR the past twenty years I've been traveling across the country, meeting women in the specialty stores that carry my products and through many interviews and live, phone-in radio and TV talk shows. My appearances generate many of the questions that have been on all our minds at one time or another. These are echoed in letters I receive and by women who recognize me on the street, in restaurants, even in the air! I'd like to answer those most frequently asked right now.

CAN STRESS HAVE A NEGATIVE REACTION
ON THE COMPLEXION?

As far as I'm concerned, stress is the most common cause of skin problems. The doctor who first said "The skin is the barometer of the emotions" is a psychiatrist. In his practice he can see how the emotions, and certainly mental anguish, take their toll physically: excessive fatigue, loss of hair and, most of all, bad skin.

Under pressure the face can break out into pimples, hives, rashes; oily skin seems to become oilier; dry skins wither. (Even happy excitement can be bad if excessive: overimbibing, rich foods and a lack of sleep can foul up the body's chemistry and cause havoc.)

The source of the stress can be almost anything that can upset you: new responsibility at work, pressure at home, a death, the loss of a friend moving away, frustration in a marriage, acne that doesn't clear, overweight that you struggle to lose. The answer is to find new ways to release the tension so that it doesn't show up on your face.

Relax.

First, concentrate on improving your mental attitude. Make decisions that are best for you—if you don't want to spend the holidays at Aunt Gertrude's, don't go. If you have more work on your desk than you can handle, don't accept any more projects—the upset at not being able to do them well will only add to your problems. Learn to block out all external influences for ten minutes each day, whether you go into your bedroom for a short nap, close the door at your office or simply take a walk without having to run any errands.

Second, look for a physical release through exercise. Anger, frustration and stress leave your system with the energy output needed for a set of tennis or calisthenics. Exhale the tension with every breath during the exercise.

Third, learn to distinguish between the different types of stress and how to cope with each. Recognize those situations which bring on unwarranted stress; perhaps it's your inability to say "no" to the requests (or demands) of others that keeps you from doing what you want to do. Stop such situations before they can have a chance to happen.

When it's a self-imposed stress, such as taking on extra work to advance your career, think of it as dynamic stress: positive and self-enhancing—and live with it.

Some stress is unavoidable, as when a loved one dies. Try to work it out of your system; accept it as a time of grief that must be lived through. Relax, knowing you can't control it, only temper it. It may sound trite, but stress that is properly handled can help you grow as a person.

CAN ANYTHING BE DONE FOR ACNE?

First ask yourself if what you have is really acne. Occasional break-outs aren't severe acne, especially if they are spot occurrences. One pimple can be due to a variety of causes: the water you're drinking in a new city, the food you eat on vacation (cooked in local water), the air you're breathing in that new location, a new makeup (oil/creme-based products can clog a pore, particularly if you're not cleansing thoroughly), any stressful situation. (NOTE: Stress can turn blackheads into blemishes if you let your nervous fingers pick at them and break the skin, and then into scars if you pick again at the scabs that form. Don't let stress get the upper hand—either one of yours!) Leave the "spots" alone. Improve your cleansing, increase rest and exercise. Skin often clears itself with no help from you.

More problematic are frequent break-outs in conjunction with oily skin. The face and back are the common target zones because these areas are blessed (a mixed blessing) with the greatest concentration of oil glands, and overactive oil glands are a large part of the acne problem. Oil production is triggered by hormones, and as hormone levels change, the quality of your skin may change, too. Hormonal activity seems to peak in adolescence, explaining why teens suffer the most. It declines in old age, but often medication taken in later years can affect hormonal changes that can cause break-outs all over again!

There are three oil-based skin conditions that can exist separately, or in any combination, on various areas of the face, primarily the T-zone. Only the third is acne.

1. *Excess oiliness.* When the oils you produce are thin, they rise to the surface and spread across your face. You may feel greasy, but there is a bright side: pores aren't clogged and this lubrication will stave off lines for quite some time. Cleanse well two or three times a day, and blot off excess oil with a tissue in between (excessive cleansing seems to stimulate the oil—four times a day is too much).

2. *Clogged pores.* When the oils aren't thin enough to reach the surface through the pores, they can become trapped within these passages (blackheads), or lodge under the skin (whiteheads).

Blackheads are not always noticeable; you may only *feel* them as you cleanse. But if your pores are enlarged, you may see the blackened tips of these clogs, colored from the oxidation of the hardened oils as they reach the surface openings, not from dirt. Squeezing blackheads has two drawbacks: breaking and bruising the skin surrounding the clogged pore and the inability of untrained hands to remove the whole clog (the area can become infected, causing a worse blemish). Let your cleansing and dermabrasing clear pores gently. If your blackheads are profuse, see a dermatologist about having them correctly removed.

Never try to remove whiteheads yourself. Called *white*heads because of their pearly appearance, the clogs are the result of oils mixing with other body fluids; trapped *under* the top layer of skin they don't oxidize as do surface clogs and must be carefully drawn out by a professional if your at-home program doesn't do the job.

3. *Pimples and pustules.* These are the real troublemakers; they brew under the skin for days at a time, driving you nuts. Trapped oils and body fluids are mixing under the skin so that instead of a blackhead you have a sore, reddened accumulation trying to burst through. When they reach the surface, they are filled with pus and look and feel as though the skin has erupted. This is not a skin condition you can cure at home. A dermatologist can prescribe anti-inflammatory medication and help you avoid acne scars.

What causes break-outs? I'm often asked. If we knew that, there'd be no more acne! Yes, hormones and oil glands contribute, but there's no way to fully regulate them *yet.* There are other contributing factors that can turn oiliness into disaster. Being alert to them can help keep your skin under control.

Sluggish skin. Lazy skin doesn't release oils readily; they get trapped in pores. Revitalize your skin with gentle dermabrasing.

Diet. A poor one can mean skin that isn't healthy enough to fight break-outs. Though most doctors have given all foods except those containing iodine (shellfish, spinach) a clean bill of health, chocolates, sodas and the like don't contain anything to enhance skin. If they're not helpful, they can be harmful.

Stress can trigger biological changes in the system that set off the break-out syndrome. If you don't master it, stress will never leave you— neither will the pimples. The loss of sleep (stress keeps you up at night) worsens the situation.

Medication has been known to bring on break-outs. Tranquilizers, diet pills, pep pills, birth control pills—all can affect the skin.

Hair that swishes across your face, especially bangs, adds to the oiliness. Facial hair along the jawline can aggravate clogged pores, too; oils cling to the hair shafts, fester in the pores.

Makeup, if of a heavy consistency, can cause blockage in the pores that will turn into pustules to be released.

At the dermatologist's. A qualified doctor will remove pus-filled pimples and blackheads without breaking the skin. The dermatologist can also prescribe antibiotic pills or lotion (for the allergic patient) to help curb inflammation. It must be said that these medications have only limited effectiveness, and varying degrees of side effects, just like any other prescription. But the help they provide can make a lot of difference.

New therapies are being developed to further lessen acne's severity, and its resultant discolorations and scars. But it is still a matter of controlling acne—immunizations against acne are still not available.

WHAT IS THE DIFFERENCE BETWEEN AN ALLERGY AND A SENSITIVITY?

There is a wide spectrum of tolerance to irritants, from those who can withstand almost anything to those who will react negatively to almost everything.

Sensitive skin is fragile skin; it breaks and bruises easily, heals slowly. A sensitivity shows as a nearly instant, topical reaction to an irritant and can affect many people.

Allergy-prone skin can be oily or dry, hardier, too. An allergic reaction follows an incubation period of twelve to twenty-four hours or twenty-four to forty-eight hours and occurs only in people who are disposed to react to a particular chemical or substance. In the case of an allergic reaction to a food, the body produces certain substances as a result of the digestive process, and one of those substances precipitates the rash.

To ease either problem, it is important to locate the source of the irritation and to stay away from it. Because sensitive reactions occur so quickly, it's easy to tell if it was the ammonia you just used in the bathroom or the depilatory you put on your legs. You should, however, test every product to be used on your body before applying it liberally or to your face. Do a patch test on a small area of the inside of your right arm to avoid having an obvious reaction, should you develop one. Leave the product on for twenty-four hours. Should any redness or itching occur, don't use it again.

Allergic reactions are harder to attribute to a source. In the day or two it takes for the reaction to surface, you might have eaten a dozen foods, worn three changes of clothing and been exposed to a handful of allergens. A dermatologist or your family doctor will be needed to isolate the culprit. He will compile a family history of allergies and test you for reactions to a dozen or so of the major causes. Tests are often done on the back because it is a large, flat area easy to examine. Always make specific notes each time you have a reaction to find a common denominator: wool sweaters, a fruit, a creme-based lotion.

Two sources of allergens:

Cosmetics. Not only women but more and more men as well are developing allergies, as they begin to use many products previously reserved for their wives. Buying products labeled "hypo-allergenic" is not really a protection. Almost all companies have removed as many

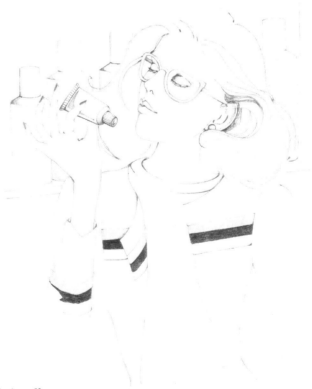

Scrutinizing labels for allergens.

known potential irritants as possible. Allergies can result from the more indispensable ingredients and can be cumulative: the use of two or more products containing a common ingredient which acts as an irritant can combine to cause the allergic reaction. Ask your doctor to test you for any you suspect. Look for the common denominator on labels of all your products and find replacements that don't contain it. (Labeling has been a great help to the allergy-prone, and companies concerned with the consumer's well-being have readily complied with the new legislation requiring it.)

Fragrance is often the culprit. But don't confuse a scent so heavy it repels you with a scent to which you have an allergic reaction. And being allergic to one scent doesn't mean you are allergic to all. The irritant might be only one of the many essential oils. Unfortunately, perfumers are most afraid of letting others in on trade secrets through labeling and try to get around the law, so that cross-checking labels isn't always easy. The irony is, of course, that there are more fragrance-related allergies than those associated with skin-care products.

Research is ongoing. Recently I was at a symposium for dermatologists and manufacturers of skin-care and makeup products intended to bridge the gap between us; we discussed the most prevalent allergies and the ways cosmetics can circumvent them. It was a positive exchange of information and a source of encouragement for the allergy sufferer.

Unfortunately there are skin reactions that not even the most qualified doctors can cure. About fifteen years ago I was plagued by a condition known as urticaria, or giant hives. As suddenly as could be, I broke out—and for no apparent reason. I was given every imaginable test at more than one medical center, and the cause was misdiagnosed more than once. One doctor asked if I had been eating anything out of the ordinary. I remembered having pork at a Polynesian restaurant. "Ah!" he said. "A classic case of trichinosis." Tests were done at the poison-control center in Atlanta, and it wasn't that at all. He had, however, given me a scare: food poisoning can be fatal.

In the hope of locating the cause for these hives which would disappear and then pop up at any moment, I stopped using all manner of makeup, fragrance and nail polish. I stopped drinking liquor, and I eliminated all sorts of foods. Once I was so frantic that Hal and I moved our family into a hotel for the weekend to see if it was something in the apartment—the fabric of the drapes, a plant—to no avail. I did everything I could think of—I even went to visit my father in Florida, leaving Hal and the kids behind, in case one of them was the culprit! The condition lasted for three years, on and off, until, as suddenly as the hives started, they stopped. The cause was never found.

It was an absolutely terrible period for me. What was so heart-breaking was the hives' unsightliness. With all the public appearances I had to make, I worried constantly about break-outs. The condition was so limiting! About the only medical explanation that made sense blamed the hives on stress. I can honestly tell you that the anguish I felt over the first break-out was enough to prompt all the rest! What got me through these years was telling myself it was a case of mind over matter —I had to stop the condition from getting to me. I relaxed as best as I could by repeating the Serenity Prayer: "God grant me the serenity to accept the things I cannot change, the courage to change the things I can and the wisdom to know the difference." A copy of the prayer sits on my night stand so I see it first thing in the morning and the last thing at night—my own form of meditation.

ALLERGY ALERTS

- On vacation, even in this country, always drink bottled water. In Houston, for instance, the tap water seems to have twice as much chlorine as in most other cities. That can cause an allergic or sensitive reaction.
- Be aware that the facial complexion can react differently from the skin of the rest of the body. Your hands may tolerate perfume, but if if you touch them to your face, and your face isn't tolerant, you can have an allergic reaction.
- Use lined rubber gloves to protect hands and arms from harsh chemicals when cleaning. These can cause irritations on even the most resistant people.

CAN THE WEATHER AFFECT MY COMPLEXION?

Yes!

Oily skin areas shine more in *hot weather* because heat liquefies the oil in the pores and the sweat spreads it more readily. Break-outs can worsen if perspiration mixes with clogged pores to form blemishes. **Be** doubly conscientious about cleansing.

Skin loses moisture as it's exposed to *dry air*, whether outdoors or due to the indoor effects of steam heat in winter, air conditioning in summer. Dry skin suffers immediately, turning red, dry and taut, itchy, flaky and lined. Add to dry air *cold, raw winds,* and you simulate the rays of a scorching sun. Overexposure causes redness and chapping in as few as ten minutes, while you wait for the bus or walk to the mailbox. In extreme weather, switch to a richer moisturizer, regardless of your age, if you need the added lubrication. After being outdoors, remove makeup and cleanse thoroughly. Apply your night creme for ten minutes; let skin fully absorb it.

Dry heat is as damaging as the cold to dry skin. Protect accordingly. Always follow the indications for skin care when engaged in sports or other outdoor activities (see page 89).

Freezing winter temperatures combine with the sun's rays, reflected by snow and ice, to cause frostbite—sunburn's winter cousin. Mild cases result in redness, swelling, even peeling. More severe exposure causes blisters—see your doctor. Recent discoveries show that steady, controlled rewarming of the skin is the best way to prevent permanent damage. Cover exposed areas of the face with your palms for warmth until you get back inside; don't rub snow into skin. For preventive protection, use a wool face mask over your moisturizer.

WEATHER ALERT IN THE FOLLOWING CITIES

· Dallas, Houston, El Paso, Phoenix, all areas of the dry desert are notorious for extremely high temperatures and extremely low humidity. Visiting there in hot months, I can't even go out during the day for any length of time. Worse, the air conditioner that cools you off dries you out even more. Invest in a humidifier; use it every night to add moisture to the air. Wear moisturizer as soon as you're old enough to ask for it; wear it around the clock, even if you're staying indoors.

· Denver, Aspen, the cities of the snow belt: Protect against the sun's reflection on snow with sun products and the 20-degree changes in temperature, and the cold winds with moisturizer and a good night creme faithfully used.

· Palm Springs, Palm Beach, Miami, the East Coast/West Coast sun belts: Guard against overexposure all year round. Don't major in sunning (take frequent trips north!). Chapter 5, The Tan Commandments, has your name on it.

· Seattle, San Francisco, London: Damp chilly weather means an increase in humidity, great for dry skin. (Dress warmly to seal out bay breezes.) But indoors, avoid steam heat or use a humidifier.

· New Orleans, San Antonio, river cities in the South: Damp heat is good for dry skin, unsettling for oily areas of the skin. Keep skin comfortable with cold water compresses at midday. Blot off excess oils between cleansings.

- Chicago and all other windy cities: Protect against chapping from high winds; keep warm against the cold (remember the wind-chill factor means that the temperature takes a nose dive). Nourish after every exposure.

WHY IS MY SKIN DRY AFTER A FLIGHT?

It used to be that only flight attendants suffered the consequences of air travel. But with everyone flying off somewhere these days, on vacations as well as on business, almost all women, and men, too, feel the drying effects of a long flight.

The reason for this is simple. As soon as the cabin doors are closed and the air pressure is stabilized, all moisture is pulled out of the air in

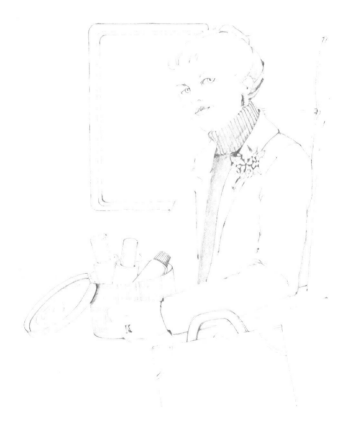

the jet. Beverages are always served on flights longer than thirty-five minutes to compensate for the body's loss of moisture. Body fluids normally lost through usual processes can't be replaced through breathing since there's no moisture in the air.

Flight attendants and pilots still have the worst skin damage: for every year they fly on the big jets, the DC-10, the L-1011 and the 747, their skin ages the equivalent of two and a half years of normal exposure. British Airways spent millions of dollars trying to overcome the problem, but found this impossible to do without upsetting cabin pressure. Since we can't fly any other way (as of yet), I found that extra skin care, in flight, helps. (Today, I'm a consultant to many of the major airlines, working with their personnel to help counter the advanced aging effects.) Follow these suggestions during your next flight:

1. Pack bottled water in your carry-on tote—much better for you than coffee or liquor—to keep skin hydrated and limit the chemicals your body is forced to ingest. Drink it throughout your flight.

2. Carry an unbreakable tube or bottle of moisturizer with you and apply mid-flight and once again before landing. Use it on your face and your hands, anywhere skin is exposed. Avoid wearing face makeup during the flight—your skin is dry enough without heaping on makeup's drying effects, too. If you want to arrive looking your best, apply what makeup you need after your second in-flight moisturizing. (The moisturizer not only acts as a surface barrier against moisture loss on the plane; it also protects against climate changes at your destination, too.)

WHAT IS THE BEST WAY TO REMOVE FACIAL HAIR?

Excessive facial hair, whether on the sides of the face, around the jawline or above the upper lip, can detract from your looks.

The simplest way to remove hair is by using a depilatory, but most sensitive skins react adversely and can be reddened or irritated by the chemicals the product contains. Always do a patch test on the inside of your arm before trying it anywhere else.

Waxing is quick, but must be done by a professional, at least at first, so that you understand the procedure.

Though electrolysis is at times painful, some small areas of the face can often be de-fuzzed in one visit. The hair is permanently removed within each pore opening—a boon to those whose facial growth complicates oily skin.

Bleaching is, surprisingly, still popular, but it has two drawbacks: first, the bleach can irritate the complexion; second, the hair is still present—if the growth is thick, it will be almost as obvious as if you hadn't done anything.

CAN MY SCALP AND HAIR AFFECT MY COMPLEXION?

The scalp is a continuation of the complexion. It is still skin, though hidden under your hair. Chances are if you have oily patches on your face your scalp will also be oily, and the hair will pick up that oiliness and seem oily too.

NOTE: Hair itself does not produce oil. Hair is actually dead matter —the living part is within the scalp. Hair does, however, gets its nourishment from the scalp. If your scalp, like your complexion, is dry, hair will appear dry or brittle because it hasn't been supplied with any oil and therefore has no sheen.

Because your hair comes into contact with your face, at the hairline if short, at the jawline and across the forehead too, if longer, hair needs care, just as your skin does. How often you shampoo depends on the amount of oil your hair picks up—the more oil, the more dirt it attracts. You can shampoo every day if you need to, but once a week is the minimum. Use a mild shampoo—you can dry out your hair from harsh detergents, especially at the ends where the oils seldom reach.

TO SHAMPOO:

1. Brush hair to remove any tangles.
2. Wet thoroughly to remove as much surface dirt as possible.
3. Lather lightly. Not too much shampoo is needed if you wet hair well. Add more water, not shampoo, for better lather.
4. Rinse thoroughly, more than you think necessary. Condition if you need it.
5. Blot dry with a towel. Let your hair finish drying naturally whenever possible. Too much heat from a dryer and rollers can "sunburn" your hair.

Protect your hair against sun exposure with a tightly woven hat or scarf. Rinse out salt water or chlorine after every swim. Treat hair gently when wet; it's weaker, more susceptible to damage.

For serious scalp problems, like persistent dandruff, flaking or psoriasis, see your doctor. You can't cure these at home any more than you can solve severe acne on your own.

IS EVERYONE SUSCEPTIBLE TO SKIN CANCER?

Yes, although those with light skin and hair are the most prone. Children are susceptible as well. They can't tolerate the sun as well as an adult can; damage to their skin is long-lasting and cumulative: excessive exposure during childhood can precipitate skin cancers in later life even without added exposure. Sunblocks are excellent for inhibiting the growth of cancers by blocking out the sun's radiation.

Artificial radiation can contribute to their formation, too. There are many instances of people who received X-ray treatments for acne some thirty years ago who then developed cancers in later years. Thank goodness that form of acne therapy is no longer in use.

Moles, those brown, raised growths often called "beauty marks" can become cancerous. Some people are born with them, others develop them later in life. Always have your doctor check any new growths and any changes in birthmarks, too. He may want to have them removed as a precautionary measure.

While you are being treated for skin cancers, don't neglect the rest of your face and body. More than ever, you need protection. See page 92 for more information.

DO FACIALS AND FACIAL EXERCISES DO ANY GOOD?

I know that facials feel good, but as for doing any good, I doubt it. And facial exercises that manipulate the face and stretch the skin have to be bad.

You can't count on a facial to remedy the lack of daily skin care any more than you can count on a vitamin to make up for poor eating habits. And the thirty dollars you spend on a monthly facial is put to better use on three or four products that will help you a little more on each of those thirty days.

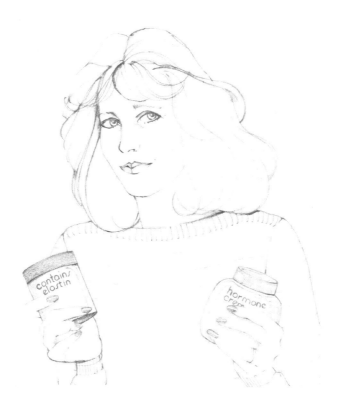

DO I NEED A CREME WITH COLLAGEN? HORMONES?

Collagen, elastin, hormones—they are all a lot of mumbo-jumbo, gimmicks loved by those who love to make a fast buck. Do you know what the source of collagen is? Cows! (Of course, this substance is found in humans, too, but I don't know of any willing donors.) I haven't seen any significant results from testing to show that it is worthwhile to use this substance in any of my cremes and moisturizers. (See page 165 for the aftereffects of X-ray treatments prescribed before adequate testing had been done.)

My father never believed in using any hormones or steroids in his original formula, which has stood the test of time—he had been using it successfully years before I started manufacturing it commercially. I don't intend to start using these ingredients now.

Yes, prescribed hormone drugs do have an effect on the body when ordered by a doctor and taken internally. But the level of hormones the FDA permits in products is so low that their presence couldn't make a difference—that's for the protection of your health. For the protection of your bank account, stay with products that have proven they work.

I KNOW THAT A FACELIFT WON'T REMOVE SURFACE LINES. CAN CHEMICAL DERMABRASION SMOOTH THEM?

Chemical peels, cryosurgery in which the skin is frozen with nitrogen and peeled off, dermabrasion in which a little, fast-moving wire brush removes layers of skin—all these procedures, based on excessive peeling back of layers of the skin to expose new, smooth skin— are dangerous. When you peel the skin down to the dermis, you expose skin that's not ready to be seen, not equipped to brave the elements. And one wrong move leaves you damaged for life: once you alter the dermis, you alter the surface appearance of the skin. Fine if it works, but if not . . .

On the other hand, dermabrading with caution, not going too deeply during this surgical procedure, really accomplishes little. It seems to me a no-win situation. (Again, this procedure is not to be confused with my dermabrase system of gentle skin sloughing.)

These techniques have been used on everything from scars to acne pits to surface lines and with such questionable results that taking the chance isn't worth it.

WHAT CAUSES/CURES BROKEN CAPILLARIES AND VARICOSE VEINS?

Both situations involve the ingrowth or constriction of blood vessels.

Broken capillaries result in thin, spidery red lines that lie close to the skin surface—the thinner the skin, the redder they seem. Very often the sun is the culprit. The capillaries are the result of sun damage—part of the skin's strategy to protect itself. Skin that's rubbed too harshly can also engender this condition. They can be removed by a dermatologist— the blood is drawn out painlessly with a needle, if the capillaries are isolated. A profusion, causing red, blotchy skin, can be camouflaged with makeup.

Varicose veins result from the breakdown of blood-vessel valves or links, causing parts of the veins to become obvious. This is often due to a poor circulation: too much sitting or standing still during the day, tight shoes and elasticized stockings or knee-high stockings. Walk more frequently, and once or twice during the day take the pressure off your legs by elevating them. Unsightly varicose veins can be removed by a doctor.

These are the questions I am most often asked. As you can see, the more serious skin woes need the attention of a doctor or dermatologist. If you have an unusual skin problem, never neglect it. Get medical attention right away.

PART IV

Skin Beauty: A Family Program

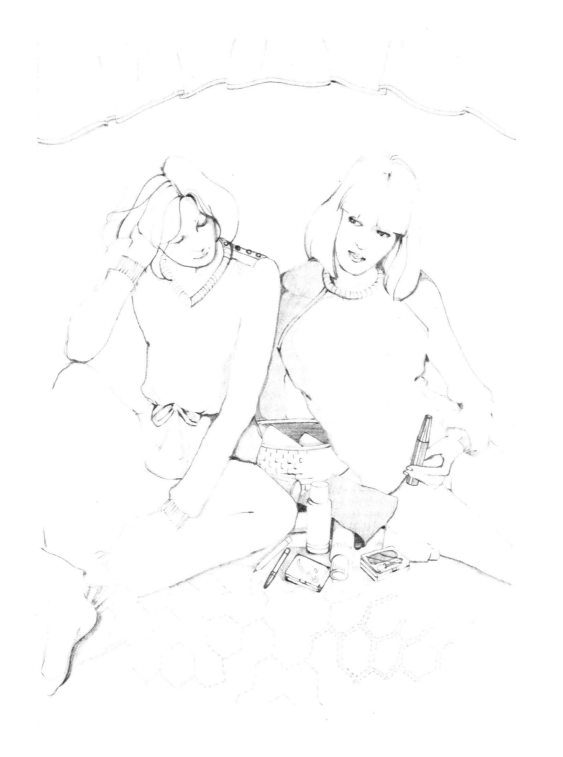

CHAPTER 10

Fresh Face:
Care for Young Beauty

I REMEMBER starting my daughter Stacey on her skin-care plan with castile soap and plenty of fresh water when she was just a little girl. Today she's fifteen and knows as much about beauty as her mother—maybe more. Skin-care awareness begins at a very early age for today's kids. Girls become interested at about the age of ten, when they start reading preteen and teen magazines. TV, too, exposes them to the glamorous world of beauty (some commercials have even gone too far: let's not rush their adulthood). Our daughters start wearing makeup sooner too, making it all the more important that they know the difference between applying cosmetics and really taking care of their skin. Because little girls love imitating their mothers, even before they know what it is they're imitating, we have to set the right example from the beginning.

When Stacey would see me taking care of my skin, she would ask about my cremes and lotions. "Would this be good for chapped lips?" "Can I put this on so I won't get sunburned?" I told her which creme to use for what and even gave her her own jars. She was so pleased to feel grown up that she made up her mind to use them and was proud of herself when she looked her best.

STACEY: I think I was eleven or twelve when I first thought about looking pretty—that's stronger than just wanting to wear makeup, which is more like a toy at first. Sure, I tried on all my Mom's stuff, but it wasn't until I was thirteen that I wore any makeup in public.

Mom taught me how to use lipstick and eyeshadows, but she also showed me how to take it all off when I was finished experimenting, and even more importantly, when I put it on for real. One of the worst things you can do is sleep with makeup on. It gets into your skin, in your eyes—and all over the pillowcase.

STACEY'S SKIN-CARE STRATEGY

Every Morning

I wash my face with a cleanser and pat dry. I use a moisturizer, especially in the winter—washing can remove some of the skin's moisture, but if you put back the oil seal, there is no better way to cleanse.

I put on a light makeup if I'm going to school, none if I'm going to be exercising. Even with getting dressed, I'm done in about ten minutes.

Every Evening

I cleanse to remove all my makeup, especially around the eyes. For stubborn mascara or liner, I use my Mom's creme remover—it's extra important to have a remover that's non-irritating. I always finish with a cold-water rinse; it takes the place of those "fresheners."

Two or Three Times a Week

I dermabrase my face to make up for the week's activity. I swim a lot, and the chlorine in the pool can really sap your skin. I like to gently clarify my complexion to compensate.

Once a Week

I use a mask, like my Mom's "Instant Acting" Face Mask—it foams into the skin and is washed off after three minutes. It's fun to use and really perks my skin tone. Great before a special evening.

Things I Never Do

1. Use any high-alcohol product, like a clear liquid cleanser that doesn't call for water, or an astringent. You have to be so careful with them because they can really dry out the skin, especially if you need to cleanse three times a day. A sudsing liquid and water is better for even the oiliest skin.

2. Touch my face with my hands unless I'm about to wash my face, and then only after I've thoroughly washed my hands. Trouble starts when you get into the habit of touching your face a lot, feeling around for break-outs or causing them by squeezing something you think is a blackhead. I even keep myself from resting my chin in my palm—that stretches the skin too much.

IRMA: I told Stacey she'd have to wash it off or it would ruin her face. The idea stuck, and she's had virtually no problems. That means a lot to a teenage girl.

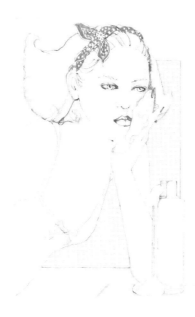

A foaming mask can be fun.

STACEY: My friends and I agree that having clear skin and keeping it clean is number one on the list, our first priority. Makeup comes second. In fact, if I had to choose, I'd rather have good skin than be able to wear cosmetics—there's just no way to hide a zit.

IRMA (*on oily skin and teen break-outs*): You don't realize it now, but oily skin is fortunate skin; it doesn't develop lines as easily as dry skin because it is kept moist. If you take proper care of it, you can control the oils now, the lines later.

Oiliness is easily washed away: use a gentle foaming cleanser three times a day; otherwise follow Stacey's example and keep hands away! Of course, even if you're careful break-outs *can* happen. But because they are very prevalent in teen years, you shouldn't be self-conscious. It happens at one time or another to almost everyone. Boys are especially prone and their acne can worsen because of shaving needs.

Superficial break-outs, not deep pustules, seem to zero in on all kids, and even adults, at one time or another. The bad thing is, compared to real acne, they're a lot like the common cold—harder to cure than pneumonia, but a lot less dangerous.

If you feel that you have a serious problem—one that doesn't go away on its own or with a little care—you can make yourself feel a lot better by getting professional help. Visiting a dermatologist can be the greatest spirit-booster; just knowing someone else is on your side can relieve a lot of stress. But not even acne can be cured; it can be helped by medication (avoid tetracyclines until age fifteen as they can cause yellowing of the teeth), consistent, gentle care and the proper attitude.

It's important to keep a cool head when facing acne. You have to talk yourself out of being upset. Anguish can only worsen the problem: you don't sleep well, your body gets run down, you get tense and start picking at your face. Take a bright outlook. Say to yourself, "I'm not going to let zits get me down!" Above all, don't let yourself become a nervous wreck—and you can talk yourself into that state as easily as you can talk yourself out of it.

Take consolation in the fact that teen years are stress-filled for your classmates too, even the ones who have clear skin: you all worry over dates, making friends, getting into college. The disasters are the same: the difference is the way you handle them.

In addition: Help yourself by drinking plenty of water—it flushes the system—and by eating a nutritious diet. There is still great dispute over food as a cause of acne. Until the final verdict is in, remember that even if it can't hurt you, nutritionless food can't do you any good either. (If you do suspect a food, rule it out for a month and see if you notice any results.) For more facts on acne and your skin, turn to page 000 in Chapter 9.

IRMA (*on the sun and young skin*): This combination is more harmful for youngsters and teens than their parents. Their tolerance level is lower, and when having so much fun outdoors, kids seem to forget about the time and protecting themselves against the sun.

Stacey was a redhead until she was five, and though her hair is closer to auburn today, she still has that fair, delicate skin that burns so easily. But fair skin isn't the only skin that needs protection—they all do. It's hard to warn a fifteen-year-old about the hazards of sun exposure —who at that age has ever believed skin can get old-looking? Twenty seems an eternity away. I found that one reason mothers are put here is to remind kids to use a sunblock after fifteen minutes and not to explain *why* until they really want to know!

IRMA (*on makeup*): The amount of money kids spend on makeup is astounding. Fortunately, they can't wear it all at once! But teen years are a great time for trying all sorts of new and different things, for experimenting and learning about their skin and their features.

STACEY: A friend and I became partners and joined a beauty club that sends us a kit filled with samples of all kinds of products, every other month. We play makeup artist for each other and then we decide what we each like best—we couldn't have so much fun alone in the cosmetic department of a large store. But not even best friends should ever share their eye makeup. This is because eye infections and diseases can be easily passed in the wand of your mascara or the brush of your eye-shadow.

When it comes to what I actually wear, I'm very serious. I use very little: no face makeup like foundation, powder or heavy rouges. I like blusher, creme in winter, powder in the summer; lipstick and a little shadow. I pay a lot of attention to my eyes and my lips, the real enhancers.

STACEY'S MAKEUP STRATEGY

Experiment
- Join a makeup club
- Try the less expensive varieties
- Buy lots of sample sizes at the drugstore: soaps, shampoos, scented talc, even colognes
- Spread the word about what you like around birthday time—tuck a note into Mom's pillow

Travel Light
   My makeup case has the following things I rely on:
- pencils: for the eyes, shadow and liner; for the lips, used with or in place of lipstick
- mascara for special occasions
- lip gloss to use alone or over pencil-colored lips
- blush

IRMA (*on makeup and break-outs*): Makeup is a double-edged sword when it comes to aggravated skin. It worsens bad skin by clogging pores and it emphasizes the slightest bump rather than concealing it. (NOTE: Zits will be less noticeable to begin with if you don't pick at them, thereby spreading inflammation, the true source of the redness.)

Makeup can work as coverage on flat scars and discolorations while you wait for them to fade. Use "treatment" makeups—those designed to work with specific problems like oiliness, pimples, dryness and the like.

IRMA (*on makeup and glasses/contact lenses*): Glasses are frequently a voluntary choice for today's girls—they can be a part of your fashion statement. But note that if you wear eyeshadow, you'll have to increase its vibrancy as the lenses tend to dim eye makeup.

If you wear contacts, you'll want to pay closer attention to eye makeup selection and removal. Choose creme shadows, as powders can flake into and irritate the eyes. Use water-soluble, not waterproof, mascara, so that any flakes will dissolve if it enters an eye. It's often easier to see your application with lenses in, but take them out before you remove eye makeup (your cleansing actions can cause one to pop out involuntarily or get filmy from the remover itself).

STACEY (*on hair care*): Your hair is indispensable to the whole picture and needs special care. I switch shampoos a lot. I love trying samples I can buy for twenty-five or fifty cents. My hair tends to be dry and frizzy, even more so after swimming, so I really need a conditioner, too. (I always shampoo/condition as soon as I get out of the pool. Chlorine has a way of penetrating even the tightest bathing cap!) I wear my hair in a simple, long, straight style, but I make sure to have the ends trimmed regularly for neatness (even if a friend does it for me).

IRMA: Oily hair needs its own kind of care: more frequent washing with a mild shampoo. If it swooshes across your face all day, it spreads skin's oil and mixes it to its own. Tie it back whenever you can.

STACEY'S HAIR CARE STRATEGY

1. Keep hair clean and, if needed, conditioned. Use mild shampoos—the newer brands contain less-harsh ingredients.

2. Brushing: a little goes a long way. Brushing dry hair can make it more brittle. Brushing oily hair spreads the oils, makes hair look oilier and dirtier. Use what few strokes you need to set your hair in place. And never brush wet hair. It's so weak then that it can break off. Separate the strands with your fingers and gently work the comb through.

3. Don't overuse hair appliances like dryers, hot rollers, curling irons. Too much heat burns and can damage the look of your hair. Twice a week is the limit. (If you shampoo more often than that, let hair dry naturally on those occasions and set in pincurls over-night—never sleep on rollers.)

4. Protect your hair from the sun—hair can get burned too. Wear a pretty scarf or a flashy hat. It's fun and safe. And if I am wearing an inexpensive brightly colored bandanna, I don't mind wearing it in the water. The sun can really damage wet, unprotected hair.

STACEY (*on diet*): I like to indulge in French fries and a cola once in a while. But ever since I started taking dance lessons and studying acting two years ago, I've become much more concerned with increasing my stamina—my physical ability—through diet and exercise.

To satisfy my sweet tooth, I make substitutions. It's always hard to say no to a milk shake, but it's easy to have a frozen banana yogurt with fresh coconut sprinkled on top instead. I love raisins, and now that I know they contain iron, I love them more. I eat them mixed with raw cashews as a great pick-me-up, or with bran and a little milk as a replacement for those sugar-coated breakfast cereals that can ruin teeth: the same number of calories, but mine has all the nutrition.

IRMA: It's amazing that our kids make these terrific choices, more so that they have all the facts needed to make them. When I was growing up, you never bothered to question the foods that were available and you certainly never dreamed that packaged foods could be bad for you.

Learning good eating habits, like anything else, is so much easier when you start early on, before you get used to having all that sugar and all that salt heaped on—leading contributants to heart disease and high blood pressure, and diabetes. (Thankfully the best baby food makers have omitted these ingredients from their products so that the sugar and salt pattern never has to begin.)

IRMA (*on overweight/underweight*): Dieting is one of our national pastimes. Very often a weight problem begins in the teens and blossoms along with you into adulthood. The teen years are, however, the best time to correct weight: young people have great willpower. That and the desire to be liked can conquer situations that sometimes even their parents can't solve.

LOSING WEIGHT

The reason people have so much trouble losing weight is that the body has regulated itself at the higher weight and resists changing. That resistance accounts for the plateaus that frequently stall dieters. The greatest difficulty comes with trying to keep the weight loss off. The brain really puts on the push to gain it back. The answer then is to diet slowly, to give the body time to adjust. Try this plan:

Week #1: Cut out all snacks, all junky foods, all sweets and double portions. Eat three average meals.

Week #2: Improve the quality of the foods you eat along the guidelines set forth in Chapter 6.

Week #3: On the fifteenth day of your diet, weigh yourself. If you've lost two or more pounds, stick with current portion sizes. If not, reduce your portions to those of my SEVEN-DAY DIET, located on p. 106, adding four 8-ounce glasses of skim milk a day.

DIET TIP: To boost your morale, keep a mental picture of you at your new weight in the front of your mind.

DIET TIP: To improve health as you lose, stay away from the usual diet foods:

· low-calorie sodas. They're all chemicals, and taste artificial. Try no-calorie club soda
· dietetic candies and chocolates. They have lower calorie counts because they are smaller than the usual ones. They are also full of chemicals, fake flavor
· canned fruits and vegetables. No wonder kids grow up hating these valuable foods. Try having them fresh, with real flavor. I think you'll like them

GAINING WEIGHT

The best way to build yourself up is through exercise. That's what puts meat on those bones and adds shape to your form. Fattening foods add fat: bumps and bulges are hardly flattering. Of course, to keep up your strength and maintain muscle, you will be able to eat more without gaining fat. The idea is to increase over-all health with the best foods. Try a fitness milk shake:

Blend two cups of low-fat milk (low-fat because you want the milk's carbohydrates and protein, not its fat content), with one large banana and one raw egg (don't worry—you won't taste it). You can add a dash of vanilla and maple syrup (the real stuff) or honey for more flavor.

Remember you can build up any area that has muscle. But neither exercise nor overeating will add inches to your bosom—this is a fallacy.

A CAUTION TO MOTHERS AND DAUGHTERS

Lately doctors have been seeing more and more cases of a disease called anorexia nervosa, an ailment that is unconsciously self-induced and most prevalent in teenage girls. Without realizing why, they starve

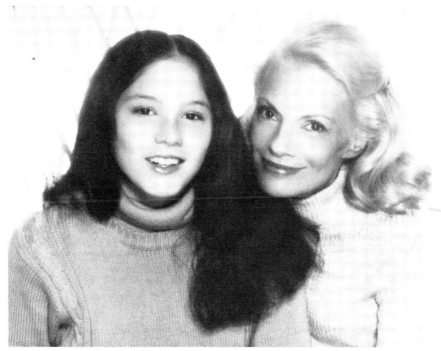

For both Stacey and me, beauty care began at an early age.

themselves, losing vast amounts of weight because they have a mental picture of themselves as undesirable, though often they are below normal weight at the outset. Without medical and emotional help, they can literally starve themselves to death.

This condition can affect an overweight girl who has reached her original goal but insists that's not enough and, as easily, the girl who has been at a desirable weight yet who suddenly sees something wrong with herself (something not physically there) and starts losing.

When overweight is a problem in your teens, always have your doctor supervise weight loss and keep good records—do so at home too, to prevent going overboard. If you notice, on the other hand, any loss that shouldn't have occurred, contact your doctor right away.

STACEY (*on size*): I'm specifically talking about height—the long and the short of it. Being a petite five feet, I've gotten my share of teasing. I found that's easy to deal with if you've accepted yourself as you are and made the most of it. Once you're comfortable with your height, others will be, too (and any teasing won't affect you any more).

STACEY (*on exercise*): I used to be so lazy that I wouldn't think twice before taking a bus, even for a distance of five blocks. But the summer before last, I started to take jazz-dancing classes three times a week as part of my acting study and it really invigorated me. Now that I'm back in school, I walk the half-mile back and forth from home twice a day and I swim as often as I can. Exercise is wonderful!

Good grooming is a must, too, especially after strenuous exercise, if you perspire a lot. It's important to shower off that healthy perspiration so that it doesn't turn into an unpleasant odor. After swimming and any exercise that calls for a sunblock, it's a good idea to wash off, too. Special products have made the job easier and more fun, and make us prettier, too.

STACEY'S BEAUTIFIERS

A *nail buffer* is great to shine up nails. I use it once a week after trimming my nails, before using a clear-gloss polish for a little dash.

A *pumice stone* is a real boost to tired feet. After a tub or shower, it smoothes calluses and removes dead skin. Afterward I dry feet very carefully (in between all toes, too) and powder them to absorb any moisture. Then I clip nails straight across.

Talc is terrific all over, before sports and after a shower—it puts a satiny finish on my skin. I carry a large container with me to dance class so that I'm never without.

After-bath splash-on cologne really makes me feel pretty. I like to use fragrance, but the heavy perfumes are out. I think that single florals for feminine types and citrusy, woodsy scents for the outdoors girl are great, and they're not too expensive either—you have to be budget-conscious when you're on a limited beauty allowance.

IRMA: It's great that our kids are so fastidious; they deserve all our encouragement. They're so aware of everything, good health, strong bodies, great personal habits.

STACEY: I'm not concerned just with looking good. Feeling good inside is very important, too. I want to do all I can to insure I always feel this way.

IRMA: What more can a mother ask for?

CHAPTER 11

About Face, Gentlemen!

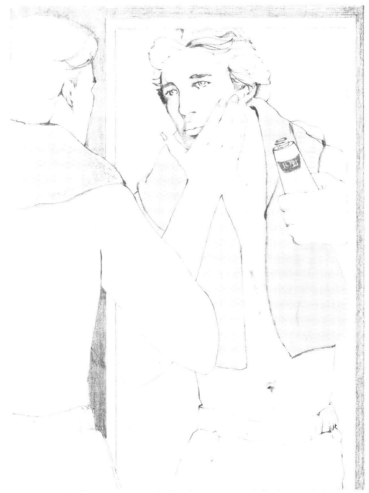

T HERE'S no doubt about it—men want to look as attractive as women do, especially today, when the world of business is fiercely competitive. There's no such thing as a woman's job or a man's job any more—except the presidency, and who knows how long that will last? Men are competing not only with women; they're also competing with younger, possibly more qualified men, too. Americans have the crazy notion that you can't look old if you're running the company. It's the direct opposite of European and Oriental cultures (a thoroughly lined face is a badge of honor to the Chinese)—but that's the way it is. And men don't want to be left out because of their looks, just as—well—just as women don't want to be considered only for theirs!

Because we recognized long before it was popular that a man's skin needs the same attention as a woman's, we came out with a skin-care line just for him. Today it's getting the wide-spread attention usually reserved for women's products because in the 1980s, men want more and more to look desirable and youthful. Isn't it about time?

Shorell for Men was the brainchild of my husband, Hal Lightman. I've turned to him for the man's-eye view on looking good.

HAL: For years, men have been told that their facial lines add character —but we know the truth. They make us look just plain old. We were at quite a disadvantage for a long time. Women got to start a beauty program as soon as they could reach the mirror, while, as teens, those boys on the baseball and football fields more than likely went unprotected against the aging rays of the sun.

We have been slowly coming out of the closet about our vanity, kept hidden until the Kennedy Administration and the youth-oriented society that followed. We began using more expensive colognes, we started having our hair "styled," rather than just barbered—my son Chip has more equipment for his hair than Irma!—and began jogging to get rid of the spare-tire-predominated cocktail-party talk. Oh, we've always been peacocks (a balding French king was the first to invent the wig!), but we were supposed to be quiet about it. Now we talk about dieting and exercising as passionately as our wives, but we still have to conquer the last frontier: skin care.

I'll be the first to admit I wasn't always keen on the idea of pampering my skin—something about its not being "manly." Irma loves to tell the story of my reluctance to encourage her to go into this business of skin care; but once I saw the results she was getting, I knew she had something. I also knew that as my wife stayed as lovely as ever, I didn't want to "mature" or look like her sugar daddy. But I wasn't sure what to do at first.

Then, during one of our visits to Florida, where Dr. Shorell lived, I asked him about this. Was there something about a man's skin that made him look so much older than his wife? No, he assured me. A man's skin is slightly thicker, but has basically the same structure. "The difference is that women care for the complexion and men don't," he said. He then explained that a man could benefit from exactly the same products. "You don't hear of male and female aspirin, do you? Well, you don't need female and male skin creme either." To prove his point, he added that his male patients had all received his now famous creme after surgery, dating all the way back to Rudolph Valentino.

If it wasn't too "unmanly" for the screen's greatest lover, I later reasoned, how bad could it be for the rest of us? This was all the incentive I needed to start using Irma's products.

I probably would have kept my "beauty" secret to myself if it weren't for a college reunion, the twentieth, some years afterward. There was a very visible difference between the way I looked and the way most of the others did—obviously not too many of them had spent the past few years using their wives' cleanser and creme when backs were turned, or going into a store for their own, all the while insisting to the salesperson that the products were for their spouse. I was asked by a few of my class members what I had been doing to stay so healthy, and I thought to myself that the results were too good to keep quiet any longer. I decided to adapt the Shorell line for men.

Today it's not only the actor who needs to preserve his looks—it's everybody from the politician who knows that charismatic appeal wins votes to the truck driver who travels through a half-dozen temperature

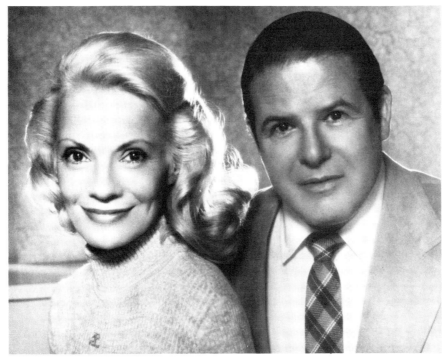

Hal and I prove that a married couple can work together happily and successfully.

changes to the construction worker who labors outdoors every day, especially in harsh climates like El Paso, Texas, where heat, dryness and the strong sun can dry skin so tight it hurts. The banker who needs to look sharp for public appearances and the business executive who knows the advantages of a youthful appearance—they need it, too.

Men don't have the ladies' back-up system of cosmetics to rely on— if you want to look good, your skin's going to have to come through for you. And that means sustained effort, just like a diet: it only works if you follow it.

If you're still hesitating, think about this: You don't find anything wrong with applying a suntan lotion in public, so why should you feel uncomfortable washing and protecting your skin in the privacy of your own bathroom? If I've learned one thing in all these years it is this: All things considered (that includes all this business about plastic surgery), you've got only one skin. You'd better make the most of it.

IRMA: Men are lucky—they can stick to a routine with very little problem. Take shaving—it's second nature to pick up that razor every morning. And what advantages you have over us: shaving removes the top layer of dead skin a little faster, promoting healthy, smoother skin sooner. It shouldn't be hard at all to improve your system. That's all you need: a little improvement.

HAL: The idea is to follow the ladies' lead and start *before* you see a problem. The reason for this is twofold: one, it's harder to correct than to prevent; two, the later you start, the more reluctant you'll be about even the slightest change.

TWO MALE MYTHS

1. You need to slap on cologne after shaving for its bracing effect.
Baloney! That habit started as a status symbol, much like acquiring a tan. Barbers would end your shave with a slap of bay rum to earn an extra tip—and they would put it on so heavily you could smell it halfway down the block. That was to make sure everyone else knew you could afford to have someone shave you.

From bay rum, we progressed to a handful of popularly priced after-shaves, the only ones available until the trend for designer scents bloomed. Today the competition among men's fragrances is almost as fierce as with women's perfume—and that's progress, *if* you put it on the right way. I'll tell you this: You won't find a woman
(continued on page 185)

applying that drying alcohol to her face. And since our skins react the same way, why should we?

After shaving, you want to soothe the face and any razor burn with a moisturizer, not sting it so bad it smarts. Save your colognes and after-shaves for below the neck.

2. *You need a dark, deep tan to be virile.*

The Marlboro man has, fortunately, gone off into the setting sun. You won't catch one of today's heroes atop a horse on a dust-beaten road, the sun blazing in his face—unless he's wearing a sunblock! The sun can only age you, especially around the eyes, where it is most damaging.

It is ridiculous to me that the serious golfer or the tennis buff or the sport fisherman will buy the latest equipment, yet do nothing for his skin, whether it's his face or his chest, his arms, his legs. All exposed skin is vulnerable to skin cancers as well as sun aging. That's not just vanity I'm talking about—it's a question of downright good health.

HAL'S SKIN-CARE STRATEGY: PRODUCTS

A foaming liquid cleanser This product should be a very effective cleansing agent without any harsh detergents; it should produce a good amount of sudsing so that you can use it as a shaving creme. I haven't used a product specifically designed for shaving in ten years—I don't like the menthol, the fragrance or the thickness of these lathers, plus they don't do anything to cleanse the face. Yet with the right cleanser such as Shorell for Men Cleansing Formula, you're not changing your routine, you're simply making a product substitution: nothing new to get used to.

A skin conditioner This product should soothe the skin, not sting like an alcohol-based liquid. It should also stop razor-burn smarting and protect against the elements. You want a sheer (invisible) lubricant with a slight firming agent to penetrate a man's skin, like my After-Shave Conditionizer.

A night preparation This product works in the evening, as invisibly as your daytime conditioner, to firm and tone the skin of the man over thirty-five. My Contour/35 for Men isn't the slightest bit noticeable.

IRMA (*on getting your man started*): It's only natural that men worry about becoming the butt of all those "night creme" jokes women have wrestled with for years. But actually, you don't have to wear your skin-care products like a mask. The best products aren't even noticeable—only the results are. And there's nothing wrong with a husband and wife knowing that both want to look their best—Hal and I often watch the news together while we wait for our lubricant to sink in.

If you can't get your husband to the store to buy skin products, treat him to them as an N.S.O. gift ("no special occasion")—75 percent of the men's treatment lines are still bought by the woman in his life.

HAL'S SKIN-CARE STRATEGY: DAILY CARE

Morning

Cleanse
Wash your hands with your liquid cleanser and rinse
Wet face with warm water
Lather face for about 30 seconds. Leave lather on

Shave
Using lather in place of shaving cream, shave as usual
Rinse off any traces of lather
Wet a face towel with warm water, wring out and apply over your face to finish cleansing pores
Rinse with cool water to close pores. Do not apply cologne or after-shave to your face or neck

Condition
Sparingly apply your conditioner to your face and neck to protect against outdoor and indoor elements

Evening

Cleanse
Wash your hands with your liquid cleanser and rinse
Wet face with warm water
Lather face for 30 seconds and rinse with warm, then cool, water
Pat dry

Lubricate
Apply your night preparation sparingly
If you've applied too much, blot after 5 minutes

SPECIAL SKIN WOES

Neck irritation: Check your laundry detergent. Some ingredients might not get rinsed out during washing and can cause an irritation, especially where the shirt creates friction against skin.

Red face: Your shirt collar probably shrank in the wash and is tighter than usual. Rinsing it in cold water and allowing shirt to dry naturally can prevent this. If the collar remains tight after the next washing, give the shirt away. The difference in comfort is worth the price of another shirt.

Stress: This is a health problem as well as a skin problem. If blood pressure is high when the pressure is on, you have trouble on all fronts. See your doctor and think about taking executive therapy: your face will respond along with your attitude.

Beards: Awfully attractive!—but they often make skin care more of a chore. Use a liquid cleanser, then a dermabrasing lotion (see pages 48–49) to penetrate to the skin surface (the applicator does a much more thorough job than fingertips). Don't neglect the exposed areas of your face, like cheeks and forehead.

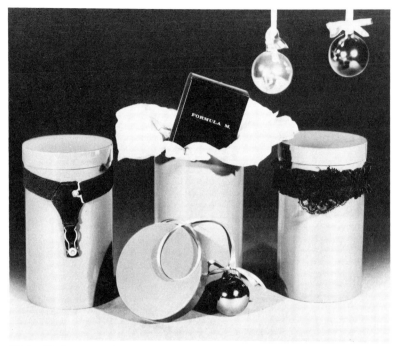

This Christmas advertising gimmick emphasized the point that my father's creme—first called Formula M7—was for men and women alike, making us pioneers in the area of skin care for men.

HAL (*to the men who work/play hard*): Taking care of your body means a little more than working out twice a week at the gym and eating right. The body needs some external care too—as the ladies say, skin doesn't stop at the neck! Give yourself a little extra attention:

In the shower. Use an abrasive sponge and cleanser to get rid of dead skin lounging around the surface. Afterward, rub in some body lotion and use talc to absorb any moisture the towel misses.

In the tub. The European influence has deemed tubs O.K. for the American male. Nothing feels so good as a five-minute soak in a foaming bath. It relieves tension and makes you forget work.

Remember, you can be as fit as a fiddle, but if you don't have a healthy appearance too, you're out of the game. (Women don't find anything sexy about dry, rough skin!)

HAL (*on cosmetic surgery*): It's an option more and more men are taking. Look at these statistics:

In 1960, one out of every six facelifts were being done on men. Today, it's one out of four.

In 1960, one out of every four eye lifts were being done on men. Today it's one out of two.

The operations are the same as those performed on women. However, the eye lift usually accomplishes much more of a change in a man's appearance—this is the area that shows most signs of age. Facelifts aren't as necessary. Hence the record number of operations in that category.

But cosmetic surgery is not like having a cola, or even spending a week at a spa. People don't always know what they're getting themselves into. To make a more informed decision, read through Chapter 8.

Ironically, when I'm on the road, promoting the Shorell for Men line, customers always want to look behind my ears for telltale surgery scars. I let them—and I laugh when I see how surprised they are that there aren't any! That's what prevention is all about.

HAL (*on discriminating against looking good*): I still take a ribbing some days about being so interested in skin care. I'm often invited to do local TV shows to talk about "men's cosmetics"—as a gag. But by the end of the program, the host and those in the studio are as hooked as I am. Let's face it, we're all getting older, but none of us wants to look it: first we joke about it, then we get down to business. Skin care is part of that business—just another extension of the jogging, the touch-ups we do on gray hair, the struggle to fit into the same size pants we did at twenty-five. The last person who you should discriminate against is yourself; why shouldn't you look good if you can?

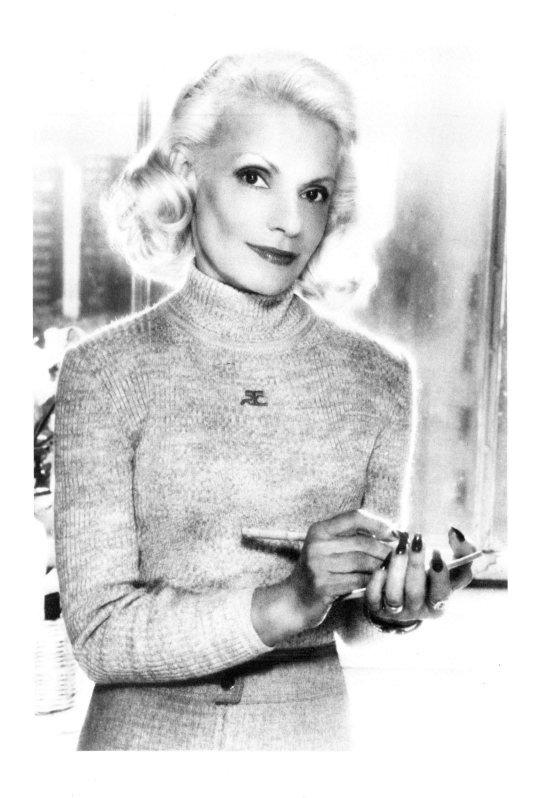